Vitamins for
Better Health

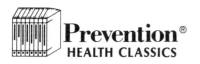

Prevention®
HEALTH CLASSICS

Vitamins for Better Health

by the Editors of Prevention® Magazine

Written and compiled by

Sharon Faelten

With contributions by

Stefan Bechtel
Mark Bricklin
John Feltman
Carlton Fredericks, Ph.D.
William Gottlieb
Jane Kinderlehrer

Jody Kolodzey
Eileen Mazer
James Nechas
Emrika Padus
Kerry Pechter
Tom Voss

Sue Ann Gursky, Research Associate

Rodale Press, Emmaus, Pennsylvania

NOTICE

If you are taking large amounts of certain vitamins, some laboratory tests may give incorrect results. Other vitamins may interfere with prescribed medication. For those reasons, it is important that your doctor be aware of any supplements you take.

Also, the information in this book is not intended as a substitute for medical treatment. We urge anyone who suspects he or she has a health problem to seek professional medical advice.

Printed in the United States of America on recycled paper, containing a high percentage of de-inked fiber.

Book series design by Barbara Field.

Library of Congress Cataloging in Publication Data

Faelten, Sharon.
    Vitamins for better health.
    (Prevention health classics)
    Includes index.
    1. Vitamins—Physiological effect. 2. Vitamins in human nutrition. 3. Health. I. Prevention (Emmaus, Pa.) II. Title. III. Series.
QP771.F33   613.2'8   81-21045
ISBN 0-87857-381-X paperback   AACR2

2 4 6 8 10 9 7 5 3 1 paperback

Contents

Introduction

Who needs vitamins?

You do. You can't live without them—literally. Every organ and tissue in your body requires one vitamin or another—and often several—for you to stay healthy and alert. Vitamin C, for example, takes part in dozens of functions, from healing wounds to building immunity. What's more, vitamins often overlap in their duties. For instance, vitamins A and C and the B vitamin pantothenate all help shield us from stress. Thiamine (vitamin B_1), niacin and B_{12} (cobalamin) each help to keep our minds sharp. No vitamin, in fact, performs one job and one job alone. All work together for the total good of your body.

Of course, it's rare for Americans to suffer from what doctors call a "clinical" deficiency of a vitamin, the type in which very little of the vitamin is left in the body and symptoms show up that a doctor can spot in an examination. But *sub*clinical deficiencies are a different story. That's the type in which *some* of the vitamin is missing; there are no outright symptoms, but the deficiency pesters you with problems like fatigue or poor skin. And subclinical deficiencies are common. Especially if you count yourself among one or more of the following groups.

PREGNANT WOMEN. "Eating for two" means that a mother-to-be needs to get enough vitamins for both herself *and* her baby.

WOMEN ON THE PILL. The B vitamins folate and pyridoxine (B_6) are often low in women taking oral contraceptives. Needs for B_{12} go up, too.

WOMEN PAST MENOPAUSE. Bones tend to thin out and break easily after a woman's menopause—unless vitamin D is there to boost calcium absorption. New evidence also indicates that vitamin K may help, too.

ELDERLY MEN AND WOMEN. As we age, we absorb nutrients less efficiently. That's a fact of life. We may eat less food, too, cutting nutrition back even further.

DIETERS. Less food means less vitamins, no matter what our age. People who cut down on meat and dairy products—prime sources of B_{12} and other B vitamins—are especially vulnerable.

COFFEE AND TEA LOVERS. Drinking coffee and tea flushes thiamine out of the body faster than diet can replace it.

HEAVY DRINKERS. Alcohol interferes with absorption of folate and vitamin A.

PEOPLE TAKING MEDICATION. Various drugs interfere with absorption of specific vitamins.

PEOPLE WHO ARE ILL OR WHO ARE RECOVERING FROM SURGERY. Recuperation puts heavy demands on vitamins A and C and several B vitamins, including thiamine. With too little of those nutrients, recovery drags.

PEOPLE UNDER STRESS. Emotional or physical stress increases our needs for several vitamins, especially A, C and the B vitamins folate and pantothenate.

CONVENIENCE-FOOD CONSUMERS. Food processing and extended storage robs food of vitamins such as vitamin C and folate. The more packaged or prepared foods a person eats, the more vitamins he may be missing.

You probably fall into one or more of those categories. And that means you need to pay close attention to your vitamin needs. And vitamins don't only help keep you free from sickness. They may also cure. In the following pages, you'll learn how vitamins can help to:

- ease the common cold;
- calm frazzled nerves;
- wipe out fatigue and headaches;
- unknot leg cramps;
- do away with forgetfulness, confusion and depression;
- clear up acne, cold sores, rashes and other skin problems;
- promote healing of cuts, burns and bruises;
- relieve asthma attacks;
- improve vision;
- cure anemia;

- remedy colitis;
- clear out urinary tract infections;
- lower cholesterol;
- quell chest pains;
- strengthen the heart;
- relieve shingles;
- dissolve premenstrual tension and other women's problems;
- overcome infertility;
- treat cancer.

There's no doubt about it: Vitamins are for better health. With their help, and this book's, you may even find yourself at your best.

Breathe Easier with Vitamin A

Ever wish you had a kind of internal gas mask to protect you against all the hazards your body encounters day after day? Cold viruses, bacteria, chemical pollutants and other airborne enemies constantly bombard your skin, throat and lungs—and eventually find their way to every nook and cranny of your body. Somehow you've got to withstand all that.

Well, you *do* have a "gas mask"—vitamin A. This special nutrient is essential for the maintenance and repair of tissues called the *epithelium*— cells that coat the body's inner and outer surfaces and protect them from life's nastier assaults. Epithelium covers all the major organs of the body (including skin, lungs, stomach, kidneys, bladder, and reproductive organs) and lines its various passageways (ears, throat and bronchial tubes, intestines and so on). Notice we said that vitamin A maintains *and repairs* epithelial tissues. That's important, because every day those cells are killed by bacteria, air pollution and other environmental invaders. And every day they grow back, as good as new. *If* vitamin A is on the job.

A Shield against Colds and Flu

For instance, consider the part of your breathing apparatus that protects you from a cold—the epithelial cells of your nasal passages and throat. Some of those cells secrete a layer of mucus, a thick substance that traps bacteria and particles. Other epithelial cells are equipped with microscopic hairs called cilia. The cilia, rooted in a second, deeper layer of mucus-secreting cells, sweep **1** the top layer *and* the germs into your stomach (where they're destroyed). But if you're short of vitamin A, the cilia can't make a clean sweep.

CURING THE COLD. If a lack of vitamin A weakens the top layer of mucus, a virus can penetrate it and infect the mucus-secreting cells below. (Scientists give these two layers one name: the mucosa.) Infected, the mucosa swells and pumps out thick mucus. And that thick mucus, while itself clogging up the nose, can also snag the top layer, stalling it. (Cilia normally move the top layer out of the nose every ten minutes, making room for a new layer.) In short, you're all stuffed up.

But don't despair. Too little vitamin A may have gotten you into the problem, and a good dose of vitamin A could get you out.

The stress of a cold robs the body of up to 60 percent of its vitamin A. "In such situations," writes Eli Seifter, Ph.D., a medical professor who has studied vitamin A, "large amounts of vitamin A are needed to replace the losses and to stimulate the immunologic responses weakened by the stress" (*Infectious Diseases,* September, 1975).

And one of those "immunologic responses," Dr. Seifter told us, is the ability of the mucosa to keep bacteria from inflaming already infected areas.

That means you need vitamin A both to protect you from and to help cure you of a cold.

An Antipollution Vitamin for Your Lungs

Without the power to regenerate their epithelial cells, our lungs wouldn't last long in the chemical potpourri we breathe as air. But even with that power, our lungs are sometimes smothered by respiratory infections and diseases that have been linked to the pollutants we breathe. How can we help keep our lungs strong and safe? Once again, with vitamin A.

NO_2—THE GAS THAT MAKES SMOG BROWN. If you've ever noticed a brownish cast to smog, you've seen nitrogen dioxide (NO_2), a destructive enemy of lung health. More likely, you've inhaled one lungful after another without even knowing it's there. Automobile exhaust contributes NO_2 to the air you breathe, and so do industrial wastes. It is contained in cigarette smoke and produced when coal or natural gas is burned for heat. So if you live in an urban or industrial setting—or commute to work there—you're probably breathing NO_2.

Laboratory tests have shown that NO_2 can damage lung tissue, producing the deteriorated state associated with emphysema.

It has been found that after exposure to NO_2, animals are more susceptible to infections of the lung. And through a chain of reactions within the body, NO_2 can form nitrosamines, potent cancer-causing chemicals.

Impressive evidence shows that vitamin A offers substantial protection against that poison gas. At the Delta Regional Primate Research Center of Tulane University, James C. S. Kim, D.V.M., Sc.D., exposed three groups of hamsters to NO_2 for five-hour periods once a week for eight weeks. The exposure, explained Dr. Kim, simulated not only city/suburban industrial pollution but also the self-pollution of a habitual smoker.

During the study, one group of hamsters ate a diet lacking in vitamin A, another ate a diet adequate in vitamin A, and the third got double doses of vitamin A. Among the first group, breathing was rapid and labored during exposure to NO_2 and their lungs were severely damaged. Many showed signs of pneumonia. And instances of abnormal cell growth—the kind that is associated with the development of cancer—were widespread.

The hamsters that received a vitamin A-adequate diet fared much better. They remained in good condition throughout the eight weeks of the experiment, with no signs of pneumonia or severe inflammation. The gas had caused damage, certainly, but lung tissue repaired itself when the animals were fed enough vitamin A. The epithelial lining, for the most part, was intact—and there were few abnormal cells.

The animals that received double doses of vitamin A survived their polluted environment equally well (*Environmental Research,* August, 1978).

In a telephone interview, Dr. Kim summed up the significant implications of his experiment: "High concentrations of NO_2 destroy the epithelial lining. With enough (or a little more than enough) vitamin A, regeneration of the lung is rapid and successful. But with a low dose this protective response is retarded—and the animal suffers."

His findings should be of special interest to commuters, Dr. Kim said, because they subject themselves to conditions much like those of his experiment. "If you commute you have intermittent exposure to NO_2. You may be exposed to urban pollution for five hours, eight hours, then you come back to your house in the suburbs, where the air is cleaner. The next day you go back to the city. The epithelium in the lung has to repair itself accordingly, after each exposure."

Vitamin A can help the lungs adapt to this less-than-perfect world, Dr. Kim said. "But a commuter who doesn't get enough vitamin A is going to suffer."

In general, the effects he observed in his lab led Dr. Kim to regard vitamin A highly as "a preventive measure" for safeguarding lung health. Even the lung problems that we associate with old age, like emphysema, may be forestalled with the early, regular use of vitamin A supplements, he speculated.

Blocking Cancer with Vitamin A

Dr. Kim's experiment suggests that the preventive powers of vitamin A extend even further than that: By discouraging the formation of abnormal cells, vitamin A may protect against cancer. A number of other studies on vitamin A and lung health point to the same conclusion.

E. Bjelke, Ph.D., a scientist from Norway, gathered data on 8,278 representative Norwegian men, including detailed information on their smoking habits and eating habits. Analyzing dietary questionnaires, Dr. Bjelke estimated their vitamin A intake. Then, five years later, Dr. Bjelke conducted a follow-up survey. He found that 38 of the men had developed lung cancer. And there was a pattern to who had gotten cancer and who had not. To put it simply, men whose diets provided a lot of vitamin A were significantly less likely to develop cancer than those who took in a little (*International Journal of Cancer,* vol. 15, 1975).

In a more recent study of 16,000 men in England, those who developed cancer, especially of the lung and digestive tract, consumed significantly less vitamin A-rich foods than a healthy control group (*Lancet,* October 18, 1980).

Skin Needs Vitamin A

Skin, too, is an epithelial tissue. And vitamin A helps keep it healthy and fresh.

"Vitamin A is a must for the correct maturation and growth of the skin from its basement layer," explained Carl Reich, M.D., of Alberta, Canada. "The basement, or bottommost layer of skin, is stronger and healthier with vitamin A. That layer eventually moves to the surface as skin cells die and are sloughed off. Since the layer is stronger, it lasts longer—it doesn't become scaly and dry and rip off too soon.

"I give vitamin A all the time to clear up dry skin," Dr. Reich told us. "It's like fertilizing the lawn. The skin grows better!"

Max Vogel, M.D., also from Alberta, uses vitamins A and D to treat dry skin. "I usually give A and D vitamins in the form of halibut- or cod-liver oil," he said. "Taking a fish-liver oil supplement two or three times a day helps dry skin."

A AND E FOR ACNE. Dry skin isn't pretty, but acne is worse. It usually occurs on the face, with pimples and blackheads being the most obvious symptoms—symptoms that are hard to clear up. But when Samuel Ayres Jr., M.D., and Richard Mihan, M.D., of Los Angeles, gave their acne patients 100,000 I.U. (international units) of vitamin A and 800 I.U. of vitamin E, the patients "had very good results," said Dr. Ayres. And the doses of vitamins were usually reduced after a few months. (See the chapter on vitamin E for more on that nutrient.)

Save Your Sight and Hearing

Probably the best-known connection between diet and sight involves vitamin A. The retina of the eye is made up of light-sensitive cells called cones and rods.The cones are sensitive to color, while the rods are only able to detect different shadings of light. The rods contain a pigment called rhodopsin, which is a chemical cousin of vitamin A. When light strikes a rod, its rhodopsin is chemically broken down, and can be restored to working order only if vitamin A is present.

In this case, a vitamin is the very stuff from which vision is "made." If the body is lacking in vitamin A, the natural restoration of rhodopsin to working order does not take place, and the rods quit working.

NIGHT BLINDNESS. The first sign of a failure in rod function is a loss of night vision. Night vision is, of course, vision in light so dim that the eye can no longer distinguish colors, and must rely totally on its black-and-white vision. Proper night vision is totally dependent on the rods, and therefore on vitamin A.

Heavy drinkers are at special risk for night blindness, since alcohol seems to interfere with the liver's ability to store and mobilize vitamin A. In one group of 26 patients hospitalized with alcohol-associated cirrhosis of the liver, 14 had problems in adapting their vision to darkness. Daily supplementation with vitamin A helped 8 of those patients overcome night blindness within two to four weeks (*Annals of Internal Medicine,* May, 1978).

Similar results were reported by a trio of Boston researchers. In one case, a 55-year-old man had a 5-year history of progressive night blindness so severe he needed a flashlight to see at dusk. He had been a heavy beer drinker for 25 years. After taking extra vitamin A daily for four weeks, this man regained normal night vision.

GLAUCOMA is much more serious than poor night vision. Increased pressure and fluid buildup inside the eyeball can lead to total blindness. But here again, there is evidence that vitamin A may have some protective effect.

"In Europe the incidence of primary glaucoma is on the order of 1.5 percent of patients seen in an average ophthalmic practice. . . . In West Africa, the incidence is some 30 times that in Europe," said Dr. Stanley C. Evans of Ibadan, Nigeria.

"Whereas in Europe glaucoma does not usually occur below the age of 40 years," he continued, "in West Africa it occurs at all age levels from children of 8 years upward. This evidently is due to the fact that in West Africa the nutritional deficiencies responsible for glaucoma are worse than in Europe, so that not only does it occur in the younger age groups but its progress in development is also very much more rapid."

Although many factors are involved, Dr. Evans said, "Usually the precipitating cause of many eye disorders, including primary glaucoma, is a vitamin A deficiency." When he gave nutritional supplements, including large doses of A, to a group of patients suffering restricted vision, blind spots and eye pain, their glaucoma was controlled just as effectively as with conventional drug therapies. That was verified by periodic measurements of the pressure inside the eye (*Nutritional Metabolism*, vol. 21, suppl. 1, 1977).

Janitor in an Eardrum

Vitamin A plays the role of housekeeper in our ears. Richard A. Chole, M.D., Ph.D., an ear, nose and throat researcher at the University of California; Davis, who in the past has investigated vitamin A's impact on our ability to hear, has found evidence that vitamin A is necessary for the normal function of the middle ear.

"Under normal conditions," Dr. Chole told us, "mucus in the ear automatically traps dirt and bacteria and flushes it into the throat, where it is swallowed. This is how the ear cleans itself. In a vitamin A deficiency, not enough mucus is produced, and it doesn't get to the right places."

In experiments with rats, Dr. Chole found that depriving them of vitamin A resulted in breakdown of the epithelium in the middle ear. The epithelium became scaly, stopped producing mucus, and lost its ability to flush the ear clean. The result was otitis media—an ear infection.

"It is reasonable to speculate," reported Dr. Chole, "that the human middle ear undergoes similar changes to those described above [in the rat] during vitamin A deficiency. If this is the case, vitamin A deficiency may be a significant factor in the genesis of otitis media" (*Western Journal of Medicine*, vol. 133, no. 4, 1980).

In the past, Dr. Chole has shown that vitamin A does much

more than perform janitorial services in the ear. In studies with guinea pigs, he has found that the cochlea, the spiral horn in the inner ear, contains vitamin A in concentrations ten times those in most other body tissues. He has gone on to show that sensory receptor cells in the ear, similar to those in the eye that rely on vitamin A, depend on the nutrient for their hearing function.

Many People Get Too Little Vitamin A

"Vitamin A deficiency is not as rare as one would think," said Dr. Michael B. Sporn, of the National Cancer Institute. "There are groups in the United States that don't eat well, that don't get enough vegetables and milk products, which are good sources of vitamin A, and thus have marginal vitamin A intakes. For example, women trying to lose weight, living on coffee and cigarettes and junk food, are probably missing vitamin A as well as other vitamins and minerals."

According to Myron Winick, M.D., director of the Institute of Human Nutrition at Columbia University, "Both the recent ten-state nutrition survey and the young-child survey, for instance, showed that many individuals in the lower socioeconomic segments of our population have low serum [blood] levels of vitamin A" (*Modern Medicine,* July 15–August 15, 1978).

Older people, too, seem to be at special risk. A Colorado State University study of 70 women uncovered startling evidence of vitamin A deficiency. The women ranged in age from 62 to 99; some lived in nursing homes, others in private homes. The investigators found that 21 percent of the women obtained "less than adequate levels" of vitamin A from their food (*American Journal of Clinical Nutrition,* March, 1977). In that case, "less than adequate" was defined as a mere two-thirds—or less—of the Recommended Dietary Allowance (RDA) of 4,000 I.U. for women in this age group.

One reason for poor vitamin A intake may be the slow but steady change in Americans' eating habits. Normally, the vegetables and fruits in a person's diet can be counted on to supply generous amounts of beta-carotene, the vitamin A precursor which our bodies convert to vitamin A. But many Americans are eating fewer fruits and vegetables, including the dark green or yellow produce that is richest in beta-carotene. And the rise of processed meals and fast-food restaurants has accelerated the trend toward a diet low in vitamin A. A recent Pennsylvania State University survey, for example, found that 99 percent of customers at a fast-food outlet chose meals that contained less than one quarter of the RDA for vitamin A. In fact, the researchers noted, "there was no good source" of vitamin A on the menu (*Journal of the American Dietetic Association,* April, 1977).

But once you're aware of the many foods that are excellent sources of vitamin A, it's easy to plan meals that supply enough of the nutrient. (See table 1.)

Table 1
FOOD SOURCES OF VITAMIN A

Food	Portion	Vitamin A (International Units)
Liver	3 ounces	45,390
Sweet potatoes	1 medium	11,940
Carrots, sliced, cooked	½ cup	8,140
Spinach, cooked	½ cup	7,290
Cantaloupe	¼ medium	4,620
Kale, cooked	½ cup	4,565
Broccoli, cooked	1 medium stalk	4,500
Winter squash, mashed	½ cup	4,305
Mustard greens, cooked	½ cup	4,060
Apricots, fresh	3 medium	2,890
Watermelon	1 slice (10 inch diameter × 1 inch thick)	2,510
Endive	1 cup	1,650
Leaf lettuce	1 cup	1,050
Asparagus	4 medium spears	540
Peas	½ cup	430
Green beans	½ cup	340
Yellow corn	½ cup	330
Parsley, dried	1 tablespoon	303
Egg, hard-cooked	1 large	260

SOURCES: Adapted from
Nutritive Value of American Foods in Common Units, Agriculture Handbook No. 456, by Catherine F. Adams (Washington, D.C.: Agricultural Research Service, U.S. Department of Agriculture, 1975).
Composition of Foods: Dairy and Egg Products, Agriculture Handbook No. 8-1, by Consumer and Food Economics Institute (Washington, D.C.: Agricultural Research Service, U.S. Department of Agriculture, 1976).
Composition of Foods: Spices and Herbs, Agriculture Handbook No. 8-2, by Consumer and Food Economics Institute (Washington, D.C.: Agricultural Research Service, U.S. Department of Agriculture, 1977).

The richest source of vitamin A is beef liver. A three-ounce serving delivers a hefty 45,390 I.U. Yellow fruits and vegetables such as carrots, sweet potatoes, apricots, winter squash and cantaloupes are also fabulously rich in vitamin A, as are deep green, leafy vegetables such as spinach, broccoli, endive, mustard greens and kale. (The more orange the carrots or sweet potatoes, the more vitamin A they contain.) But be careful when you cook those vegetables; long cooking times tend to destroy much of the nutrient.

However, for nearly foolproof vitamin A insurance, you may want to try a supplement. Most vitamin A supplements are derived from fish-liver oil, and are available in capsule form. Because the nutrient is fat-soluble and stored in the body, you have to be careful not to take too much. (An excess can cause the same problems as a deficiency.)

The Recommended Dietary Allowance is about 5,000 I.U. Many health-conscious people take somewhere in the neighborhood of 10,000 to 20,000 I.U. Fifty thousand I.U. per day is probably a safe upper limit. But any supplement you take may help you achieve "Grade A" health.

Thiamine for Steady Nerves and a Strong Heart

CHAPTER 2

In *The Wizard of Oz*, you remember, the Scarecrow asked for a brain, and the Tin Man asked for a heart. While they were at it, they probably should have asked for thiamine (vitamin B₁) as well, because it's absolutely necessary for the maintenance of those two body parts.

The Brain Food for Everybody

Even a slight deficiency of thiamine damages the brain. Poor memory, irritability, depression, a lack of initiative, insomnia and the inability to concentrate are all symptoms of a mild thiamine deficiency—which sounds simple enough but is not. Too often those symptoms are diagnosed as neurosis or senility. Yet here's the rub: How does a person know when he is genuinely worked up over a bona fide problem and when he is simply deficient in thiamine? Unfortunately, he can't always tell. Nor can his doctor. Still, in one remarkable study, symptoms that seemed to be caused by real mental illness cleared up when patients were given extra thiamine.

Twenty people with problems like sleep disturbances, unpleasant personality changes, fevers of unknown cause, intermittent diarrhea and a lack of appetite were closely watched. As the researchers pointed out, many of these symptoms are normally called classic signs of chronic anxiety, and since the patients seemed to have no specific disease, most physicians would chalk their troubles up to "neurotic tension." On the other

10   hand, of course, while these symptoms are not life threatening, they *are* life wrecking, and the people involved were justifiably angry when conventional medical treatment failed to help. So some unconventional treatment was tried: The subjects were given vitamin B supplements, and they worked! The researchers reported that "all of the 20 patients noticed marked symptomatic improvement or lost their symptoms completely after the thiamine supplement," which in doctor-talk means, "they got better."

Another mental disturbance that has been linked to lowered thiamine levels is senility in older people. That's based on the fact that our ability to utilize thiamine slacks off as we age. Researchers compared the thiamine levels of 18 women judged senile to those of 10 healthy people. Fifteen of the 18 women had "suboptimal blood levels" of thiamine (meaning they were too low), while all 10 of the healthy people had "normal" levels (*International Journal of Vitamin and Nutrition Research,* vol. 46, no. 1, 1976). A second study maintained that the inability to use thiamine properly in old age suggests we should up our intake of the vitamin as we get older (*Journal of the American Geriatrics Society,* October, 1979).

Healthy Hearts Need Thiamine

So much for the Scarecrow and his new brain. The Tin Man's heart needs some thiamine help, too. This B vitamin appears to be a must for keeping the heart muscle strong. In one study, researchers from the University of Alabama Medical Center in Birmingham measured the daily thiamine intake of 74 people and then had the patients list their cardiovascular (heart and circulatory system) complaints. Dividing the people into a "high-intake" group and a "low-intake" group, they found that those with a low intake of thiamine had almost twice as many cardiovascular complaints (*Journal of the American Geriatrics Society,* November, 1967).

But there is even better evidence of thiamine's connection to heart trouble. When researchers compared the thiamine levels in the heart muscles of 12 patients who had died of heart disease to those of 10 patients who had died of other causes, they found that the heart patients had thiamine levels 57 percent lower than the other patients (*Nutrition Reviews,* October, 1955).

Finally, a study from Japan clinches the matter. In the ten days before their open heart surgeries, 25 patients were given thiamine supplements, while another group of patients were not. When their hearts were artificially stopped so the operations could be performed, only 10 percent of the thiamine group suffered abnormal heart spasms, while 30 percent of the other group were so affected. And when the hearts were restarted at the end of the operations, only 30 percent of the thiamine folks had spasms, but a whopping 95 percent of the other group did (*Medical Tribune,* March, 1966). From that study, it's clear that thiamine contributes to heart strength.

Thiamine Robbers

Fortunately, while thiamine does big things for us, we actually need very little of it. The National Research Council recommends a daily allotment of just a half a milligram of thiamine for each 1,000 calories we take in. As a result, the daily RDA is set at 1.0 milligrams for most women and between 1.2 and 1.4 milligrams for most men. But that raises the question: If our daily requirement for thiamine is so low, how come so many of us are deficient in it?

Part of the problem lies in the very nature of thiamine. Like vitamin C, thiamine is water-soluble, which means that we can't store it in our bodies. We must make new thiamine "deposits" each day, because we are also constantly withdrawing it. In addition, certain dietary habits make it even more difficult for us to renew our thiamine supply.

DIETING. When we reduce our intake of food, our thiamine supply may fall 40 percent.

POOR FOOD CHOICES. Most people don't eat thiamine-rich foods—even when on full rations. Thiamine is available in fairly high quantities in such foods as liver, whole grains and legumes, but many people do not eat them regularly, and thiamine is hard to come by in other foods.

TOO MANY REFINED CARBOHYDRATES. An overload of carbohydrates like sugary snacks, corn chips, white flour and white rice can short-circuit your thiamine metabolism. That's because those foods need thiamine to be digested, but, since they've been stripped of thiamine during the refining process, they don't give your body any to work with. The result is a thiamine deficit. With a natural diet, there's no problem, because carbohydrates such as brown rice and whole wheat contain lots of thiamine.

COFFEE. In a study on coffee's effect on thiamine, volunteers drank seven cups of coffee in three hours. Eight days later, they drank the same amount of water. On both days, researchers measured the amount of thiamine excreted later in the volunteers' urine. The amount was 45 percent less on the coffee day than on the water day—good evidence, say the researchers, that coffee destroys thiamine in the body. And decaffeinated coffee is no way out, they add. It's not the caffeine that destroys thiamine, but another strong coffee ingredient, chlorogenic acid (*International Journal of Vitamin and Nutrition Research,* February, 1976).

TEA. Should coffee lovers switch to tea? No. When some volunteers were asked to drink four to six cups of tea a day for a few weeks while eating a thiamine-rich diet, all of them still developed a deficiency within a week (*Federation Proceedings,* March 1, 1976).

ALCOHOL. Like tea, alcohol cuts down our absorption and use of thiamine, and most chronic alcoholics develop severe thiamine deficiencies. But even moderate amounts of alcohol rob the body of some thiamine.

OVERCOOKING OF FOODS. Thiamine is fragile, and high heat or prolonged cooking can destroy it.

CHLORINE. Many people drink and cook with tap water that contains chlorine. Some alarming evidence indicates that chlorine destroys thiamine in foods. Researchers cooked rice in both chlorinated tap water and distilled water, and then measured the amount of thiamine in the batches. The rice cooked in tap water had 36 percent less thiamine. When even more chlorine was added to the tap water, rice cooked in it contained even less thiamine (*Journal of Nutritional Science and Vitaminology,* vol. 25, no. 4, 1979). The problem is, of course, that it's not easy to avoid chlorinated water, and so you may want to guard against its effects with a B complex vitamin that provides added thiamine.

More Thiamine for All

The truth is that most of us may need more thiamine. Comparing the thiamine levels of diabetics and healthy people, some researchers were surprised to find that many people in *both* groups had low levels of thiamine. Fifty percent of the healthy people *and* the patients would have benefited from an increased intake of thiamine, they concluded (*American Journal of Clinical Nutrition,* October, 1977).

Fifty percent! Either you or your spouse? A thiamine deficiency is one of the most widespread of nutritional problems. To make sure you get enough thiamine, avoid refined and processed foods and stick to fresh foods. Organ meats, fish, green leafy vegetables, nuts, seeds and whole grains are all good sources of thiamine. (See table 2.) And when you cook those foods, take it easy. Remember that thiamine is one of the most fragile—but precious—nutrients.

Table 2
FOOD SOURCES OF THIAMINE

Food	Portion	Thiamine (milligrams)
Brewer's yeast	1 tablespoon	1.25
Sunflower seeds	¼ cup	0.71
Soybeans, dried	¼ cup	0.58
Beef kidney	3 ounces	0.43
Navy beans, dried	¼ cup	0.33
Soybean flour	¼ cup	0.27
Kidney beans, dried	¼ cup	0.24
Beef liver	3 ounces	0.22
Rye flour, dark	¼ cup	0.20
Oatmeal	1 cup	0.19
Brown rice, raw	¼ cup	0.17
Whole wheat flour	¼ cup	0.17
Chick-peas, dried	¼ cup	0.16
Split peas	½ cup	0.15
Salmon steak	3 ounces	0.15
Buckwheat flour, dark	¼ cup	0.14
Chicken liver	3 ounces	0.13
Cornmeal	¼ cup	0.12
Collards, without stems, cooked	½ cup	0.11
Wheat germ, toasted	1 tablespoon	0.11
Asparagus	4 medium spears	0.10

SOURCES: Adapted from
Nutritive Value of American Foods in Common Units, Agriculture Handbook No. 456, by Catherine F. Adams (Washington, D.C.: Agricultural Research Service, U.S. Department of Agriculture, 1975).
Introductory Nutrition, by Helen Andrews Guthrie (St. Louis: C.V. Mosby, 1979).

A NATURAL BUG REPELLENT

From time to time, we hear from people who've found that large doses of thiamine protect them against insect bites. In spite of the fact that there's been no clinical proof of those reports, doctors do sometimes recommend thiamine (as part of the B complex) as an insect repellent. The theory is that when we consume large amounts of thiamine, some of the vitamin is excreted in our perspiration, creating an odor that insects find disgusting enough to avoid. We humans, of course, can't smell it.

Riboflavin Keeps You in the Pink

Of course, it's not polite to stick out your tongue, but it is a good way to find out whether or not you need more riboflavin—or vitamin B_2, as it used to be called. If your stuck-out tongue looks normal in size, if it's a healthy pink color and feels smooth around the edges—that is, it's free of indentations made by your teeth—then the chances are that you're well supplied with riboflavin. But if your tongue has a purplish cast and seems irritated, you may be riboflavin deficient—especially if you've been unduly nervous lately or nagged by certain digestive disturbances.

And while we have you at the mirror, look for cracks at the corners of your mouth. Or lines radiating away from your lips. Or oily hair, teary, red eyes, and flaky areas of skin around your nose, eyebrows and hairline. Does your vision blur? Do you whip out your sunglasses at the first hint of brightness? All these things are signs of a riboflavin shortage. As a matter of fact, skin problems are among the first results of a riboflavin deficiency, because the vitamin is necessary for the health of the epithelial or skin-producing tissue.

But there's more. Because it combines with proteins to form oxygen-carrying enzymes, riboflavin is involved in the respiration of every single cell in our bodies. And riboflavin contributes to the complex process of blood production. Some researchers in London found that even a small deficiency of riboflavin can shorten the lives of our red blood cells (*Proceedings of the Nutrition Society,* February, 1980). That's why in a study of pregnant women, supplements of both iron *and* riboflavin were much more effective in raising low red cell counts than iron alone (*Nutrition and Metabolism,* vol. 21, suppl. 1, 1977). **15**

Very Important in Pregnancy

So along with other supplements and plenty of exercise, every expectant mother should add a good riboflavin source like brewer's yeast to her daily routine. In addition to benefits for the mother, the vitamin has a detoxifying effect on environmental pollutants and drugs which can harm an unborn child. Not every woman who took the drug thalidomide, for example, gave birth to a defective child, and it's been suggested that the babies born to mothers with sufficient B_2 were protected against the dangers of that drug.

And adequate amounts of riboflavin help prenatal mental development as well. Vitamin B_2 may not produce a genius every time, but "a number of important enzymes in the brain require riboflavin to function," said Richard S. Rivlin, M.D., of the Memorial Sloan-Kettering Cancer Center in New York City. And, he pointed out, "it is likely that a deficiency of riboflavin during a critical period of time probably would impair the normal development of the brain."

Insuring Your Riboflavin Intake

The Recommended Dietary Allowance for riboflavin is 1.6 milligrams for the average adult man and 1.2 milligrams for women. That need goes up during pregnancy and nursing. But other things also increase our need for riboflavin. Because it aids the metabolism of protein, our requirements increase as our protein intake does. And our bodies need riboflavin to convert another B vitamin, pyridoxine (B_6), into a form the body can use. So any condition that requires more B_6 increases the need for riboflavin as well. (For more on your vitamin requirements, see the chapter How Much Do You Need?)

A convenient and rich source of riboflavin is brewer's yeast. It contains at least 0.3 milligrams of B_2 in each tablespoon. Of course, many people shy away from it because of its distinctive taste. Others, however, have found that switching to debittered yeast or another brand name solves the taste problem. No matter what kind you settle on, brewer's yeast should be used liberally—in soups, stews, casseroles and baked goods. Two tablespoons of brewer's yeast added to every cup of flour in a recipe, for instance, is enormously beneficial and almost undetectable. And one popular way to down your daily allotment is with a yeasty tomato shake—a glass of tomato juice, plus a tablespoon or two of brewer's yeast and a pinch of basil or minced parsley, all whirred together in a blender.

Table 3
FOOD SOURCES OF RIBOFLAVIN

Food	Portion	Riboflavin (milligrams)
Beef kidney	3 ounces	4.1
Beef liver	3 ounces	3.6
Chicken liver	3 ounces	1.5
Calf heart	3 ounces	1.2
Beef heart	3 ounces	1.1
Yogurt, lowfat	1 cup	0.5
Broccoli, cooked	1 medium stalk	0.4
Milk, whole	1 cup	0.4
Almonds	¼ cup	0.3
Brewer's yeast	1 tablespoon	0.3
Brie cheese	2 ounces	0.3
Camembert cheese	2 ounces	0.3
Roquefort cheese	2 ounces	0.3
Wild rice, raw	¼ cup	0.3
Beef, lean	3 ounces	0.2
Ricotta cheese, part skim	½ cup	0.2
Soybeans, dried	¼ cup	0.2
Swiss cheese	2 ounces	0.2

SOURCES: Adapted from
Nutritive Value of American Foods in Common Units, Agriculture Handbook No. 456, by Catherine F. Adams (Washington, D.C.: Agricultural Research Service, U.S. Department of Agriculture, 1975).
Composition of Foods: Dairy and Egg Products, Agriculture Handbook No. 8-1, by Consumer and Food Economics Institute (Washington, D.C.: Agricultural Research Service, U.S. Department of Agriculture, 1976).

Liver, kidney and heart are also excellent food sources of riboflavin, although most people don't eat them every day. That means that other sources of the vitamin have to be added to the diet—milk, cheese, eggs, leafy green vegetables and whole grains. (See table 3.)

Keeping Your Riboflavin Healthy

Like other B vitamins, riboflavin is a fragile nutrient. Foods containing riboflavin must be handled with care. For example, some riboflavin—up to 1 percent of a specific food's supply—is lost each day that food is kept in cold storage, and that means in supermarkets, in warehouses and even your own refrigerator or freezer. What's worse, as it thaws, frozen meat leaches out perhaps 9 percent of its riboflavin along with 12 percent of its thiamine and 15 percent of its niacin, two other B vitamins. Exposing food to light and heat also destroys its riboflavin, and so staples should be protected from those conditions while in storage. For the same reason, it's a good idea to cover pots while cooking. And because B_2 is water-soluble, fruits and vegetables should never be soaked before they're used; the soaking simply washes the vitamin away. As little water as possible should be used in cooking riboflavin-rich food, and the pot liquor that remains after the process should be retained—it's rich in B_2. When soaking seeds and grains for sprouting, the soak water should also be kept for other uses.

So, if the question is whether you are getting enough riboflavin, the answer may be on the tip of your tongue. And answering it may help keep your whole body in the pink.

Niacin Limbers Up the Body and Mind

CHAPTER 4

Fortunately, very few people have a severe enough deficiency of niacin to get pellagra—a fearsome combination of symptoms that can include hallucinations and delirium. But that doesn't mean niacin should be taken for granted. A mild deficiency of niacin, according to some medical researchers, can cause such "everyday" problems as skin rashes, insomnia, irritability, headaches and arthritis. And it's no wonder that skin and mental problems erupt when niacin is in short supply. Scientists have so far identified more than 40 biochemical reactions that depend on niacin. And sensitive, vital layers of tissue in the skin, tongue, intestines and nervous system need the nutrient to stay healthy.

A Natural Tranquilizer

Psychiatrists have successfully prescribed niacin as a tranquilizer for more than 20 years. In fact, Swiss researchers compare the vitamin's effectiveness with that of the tranquilizer Valium—without the risk of harmful side effects or addiction.

Niacin comes in two forms, niacinamide and nicotinic acid, and which one you take to improve your outlook depends on your symptoms, said H. L. Newbold, M.D., a New York City psychiatrist. "People who are slowed down and depressed do better on nicotinic acid and . . . tense, hyperexcitable people do better on niacinamide.

"Keep in mind," explained Dr. Newbold, "that while most people feel better within days of beginning a niacin regimen, some require months to feel the benefits. It is especially important **19** to give this vitamin a lengthy therapeutic trial because its potential benefits are so great" (*Mega-Nutrients For Your Nerves,* Peter H. Wyden, 1975).

BRIGHTER OUTLOOK FOR SCHIZOPHRENICS. Some nervous problems are more than a simple matter of the jitters or depression, though. In schizophrenia, for instance, *thought* and *perception* are disrupted. But the weird thoughts and strange perceptions of schizophrenia are often the symptoms of *physical* disorders. And that means they can be healed with nutrition.

Abram Hoffer, M.D., a psychiatrist in British Columbia, was a pioneer in the nutritional treatment of schizophrenia. In 1952, he and a colleague gave niacin to eight schizophrenic patients. They immediately improved. Continuing the study, the doctors checked their patients' progress for the next 15 years. All were well 15 years later—and all were still taking niacin (*Orthomolecular Psychiatry,* Freeman, 1973).

In another study, Dr. Hoffer gave 73 hospitalized schizophrenics niacin and compared them to 98 who were not taking niacin. During the next three years, only 7 of the niacin patients had to be readmitted to a hospital, while 47 of the nonniacin patients were readmitted (*Lancet,* February 10, 1962).

STAVES OFF SENILITY. Dr. Hoffer also feels that niacin can help stop senile changes or slow them down greatly, probably due to the nutrient's effect on red blood cells. Oxygen-laden red blood cells have a "spark," a negative electrical charge. Like the negative poles of two magnets, two red blood cells will repel each other. They have to—to carry their oxygen to the brain's tissues, they must crawl single file through tiny blood vessels called capillaries. But if, because of disease or old age, the red blood cells lose their charge and bunch up, a microscopic traffic jam is created. The brain gets less oxygen. Senility—or any of a dozen other varieties of dullness and irritability—can set in. But niacin restores the red blood cells' electrical charge, sparking the brain back into working order.

Dr. Hoffer and his colleagues gave large doses of niacin to middle-aged and elderly people. Of ten people suffering from senility who got niacin, five "recovered," and two had "marked improvement." Three others did not benefit from the niacin. Four people who were normal when the therapy began remained well.

A Helper for the Heart

Doctors have long known that niacin, in the form of nicotinic acid, can help lower the level of blood fats like cholesterol and triglycerides that can muck up arteries and cause heart attacks. One such doctor—Edwin Boyle, M.D., clinical professor at the Medical University of South Carolina in Charleston—has been called "North America's foremost expert on niacin and heart disease." For good reason. Dr. Boyle has been treating heart disease with niacin for over 20 years. In a telephone interview, Dr. Boyle told us that a five-year study of over 8,000 men revealed that those who took niacin regularly—1,000 men—had 25 percent fewer nonfatal heart attacks.

In his practice, Dr. Boyle uses niacin to help those who have very high levels of blood fats. Not only does niacin lower their cholesterol levels, Dr. Boyle said, but it eliminates "sludging"—the bunching up of red blood cells that we mentioned earlier. Once sludging is gone, Dr. Boyle prescribes proper diet and moderate exercise to restore a heart patient's health. "There is a proper sequence of treatment, and niacin fits into that sequence," he told us. "People with elevated cholesterol and clinical vascular disease do as well with niacin, diet and exercise as with any other regimen."

Doctors Put Niacin to Work

Though using vitamins may mark a doctor as unconventional, Dr. Boyle is hardly alone in prescribing niacin. Take William Kaufman, M.D., Ph.D., for instance.

"When I began practicing in 1941, I found it striking that patient after patient came in with a group of symptoms which were quite similar," he told us. "They might have other symptoms besides, but in these certain symptoms, such as the lack of ability to concentrate, depression, irritability, joint complaints, excessive fatigue, bloating and intestinal complaints, there was fingerprint similarity. Many patients were easily startled so they jumped when the phone rang. A number had black and blue marks on their bodies where they had bumped into things since their sense of balance was far off.

"I began tabulating symptoms, and very soon recognized that this strange syndrome was probably a form of pellagra, or niacin deficiency, that had not yet reached the degree of severity to cause the classic combination of skin rash, diarrhea and dementia," continued Dr. Kaufman. "I reasoned that if this was a form of pellagra, then niacinamide—which had just been discovered as a preventative—might provide useful treatment.

"I prescribed niacin in very small doses at first, amounting to about 100 milligrams a day," said Dr. Kaufman. "Male and female patients would return a few days later and . . . I didn't believe it!

They looked different. They acted different. They told me that their symptoms had vanished, they felt a new zest for life. I decided to test it. I gave a few of these improved patients calcium tablets instead of niacinamide. They were unaware of the change. At the end of ten days they were right back to where they had been when they first saw me. When they resumed niacinamide treatment, they once again improved.

"But even though I had good therapeutic results with this group of patients, I wasn't satisfied with this. I wanted to have a way of measuring improvements objectively," Dr. Kaufman told us. "I needed some new standards of measurements. So I designed some simple instruments I could use to measure joint mobility, and adapted other instruments for measuring muscle strength and working capacity. With these devices I could show, for example, how niacinamide properly used was enabling people to turn their heads further, as well as move their other joints through wider ranges of motion. This showed that their impaired joints were becoming measurably more flexible as long as they stayed on niacinamide."

Get Up and Go with Niacin

A lot of people might get back their get-up-and-go just as Dr. Kaufman's patients did if niacin played a larger role in their daily diet plan. A nationwide nutritional survey conducted in 1971 and 1972 by the U.S. Department of Health, Education and Welfare found that many Americans have the clinical signs of niacin deficiency.

What's most often to blame for niacin deficiency? A glaring absence of fresh fruits and vegetables, lean meats, eggs and milk in the diet. So if you want to beef up your diet with good sources of niacin, start with liver, which is at the top of the list. Lean meats and fish are also superb sources. Whole grains, dried peas, beans, nuts and peanut butter are also good sources. (See table 4.)

If you take 100 milligrams or more of niacin in the form of nicotinic acid, you may be in for a surprise. At that level, chemicals are released into your bloodstream that widen your blood vessels, and blood rushes to your skin. That sudden increase of blood flow causes your face to turn red, hot and itchy. It's called "flushing," and it's harmless. It also fades rather quickly. And if you continue to take nicotinic acid every day in that dosage, eventually the flushing won't happen. If you'd prefer not to flush, take no more than 50 milligrams of nicotinic acid at any one time, or take niacinamide.

Either way, you may find yourself moving through life more easily.

Table 4
FOOD SOURCES OF NIACIN

Food	Portion	Niacin (milligrams)
Beef liver	3 ounces	14.0
Tuna, canned in water, undrained	3 ounces	11.3
Chicken, light meat	3 ounces	10.6
Beef kidney	3 ounces	9.1
Swordfish	3 ounces	8.7
Salmon steak	3 ounces	8.4
Halibut	3 ounces	7.2
Peanuts, chopped	¼ cup	6.2
Peanut butter	2 tablespoons	4.8
Beef, lean	3 ounces	3.9
Chicken liver	3 ounces	3.8
Brewer's yeast	1 tablespoon	3.0
Cod	3 ounces	2.7
Brown rice, raw	¼ cup	2.4
Sunflower seeds	¼ cup	2.0
Avocado	½ fruit	1.8
Almonds	¼ cup	1.3
Whole wheat flour	¼ cup	1.3
Navy beans, dried	¼ cup	1.2
Soybeans, dried	¼ cup	1.2
Kidney beans, dried	¼ cup	1.1
Chick-peas, dried	¼ cup	1.0
Dates	¼ cup	1.0

SOURCES: Adapted from
Nutritive Value of American Foods in Common Units, Agriculture Handbook No. 456, by Catherine F. Adams (Washington, D.C.: Agricultural Research Service, U.S. Department of Agriculture, 1975).
Introductory Nutrition, by Helen Andrews Guthrie (St. Louis: C.V. Mosby, 1979).

Vitamin B₆ for Women's Health

CHAPTER 5

Because of its involvement with almost every important biochemical function inside the body—from the digestion of carbohydrates and fats to the smooth handling of protein—we all need B₆ (pyridoxine). Now, however, it is becoming clear that a great many of us need it in extra-large amounts for extra-special problems, from chasing away the blues to dissolving gallstones. In fact, no other B vitamin is so likely to be needed in such great quantities.

The Pill Blamed for Low B₆— and Low Moods

It's no secret that ten million women in the United States take the Pill. It's also no secret that a lot of these women are depressed. About 7 percent, according to one study. Fortunately, a spate of research in the past decade, much of it conducted by Dr. P. W. Adams of St. Mary's Hospital Medical School in London, England, sheds light on *why* Pill users are depressed. Dr. Adams, speaking to the Fourth International Congress on Hormonal Steroids in March of 1975, laid the blame on one of the Pill's more subtle side effects—a deficiency of vitamin B₆.

Dr. Adams explained to the conference that estrogen, a hormone found in the Pill, increases the metabolism of tryptophan, an essential amino acid. But tryptophan metabolism demands B₆. As more tryptophan metabolizes, more B₆ burns up. The result? A B₆ deficiency so severe that it sometimes upsets the delicate balance of the brain's chemistry, toppling a contraceptive user into the depths of depression.

24

But there's an easy way out of those depths. Dr. Adams detailed for the conference two rigorous clinical studies that he has conducted in which supplements of B₆ restored mental equilibrium to depressed Pill users.

In the first study, 22 users of oral contraceptives suffering from depression were tested for B₆ deficiency. Out of the 22, 11 women had an "absolute" deficiency—a very severe deficiency state. Dr. Adams found that the administration of 20 milligrams of vitamin B₆ twice a day benefited all 11 women. The remaining 11 women who were not severely deficient did not benefit (*Lancet*, April 28, 1973).

In the second study, 19 out of 39 women taking the Pill and also suffering from depression were found to have absolute deficiencies of B₆. All 19, after receiving 40 milligrams of supplementary B₆ each day, improved significantly (*Lancet*, August 31, 1974).

Still another study reported that when 250 "depression-prone" women received oral contraceptives supplemented with B₆, 90 percent remained free of severe depression (*Ob. Gyn. News*, March 15, 1978).

Pregnancy Raises B₆ Needs

In 1962, a decade before Dr. Adams discovered the facts about B₆ and depression, John M. Ellis, M.D., a general practitioner from Texas, had discovered that pregnant women benefited greatly from extra B₆.

In his book, *Vitamin B₆, The Doctor's Report* (Harper & Row, 1973), Dr. Ellis recounts how high-level B₆ supplements eliminated the edema (fluid retention in the tissues) which is so characteristic of pregnancy.

But B₆ is not just for pregnant women afflicted with edema. Nausea and vomiting during pregnancy may also be due to a deficiency of B₆. Two researchers, I. Reinken and H. Grant of Innsbruck, Austria, found that women suffering from nausea and vomiting in early pregnancy were deficient in B₆ (*Clinica Chimica Acta*, vol. 55, 1974).

"*All* pregnant women have an increased need for vitamin B₆," cautioned Dr. Ellis, who recommends a daily supplement of at least 50 milligrams of B₆ throughout pregnancy. "During my clinical experience with vitamin B₆, I have attended 225 pregnant women who received B₆ therapy," he told us. "Numerous signs and symptoms appear during pregnancy that are responsive to B₆. These include painful neuropathies [nerve problems] in the fingers and hands, swelling in the hands and feet, leg cramps and hands and arms 'that go to sleep.' Most of all, B₆ is a factor in the prevention and treatment of toxemia of pregnancy [a form of poisoning that may threaten the life of the mother or fetus or both] and the convulsions of eclampsia [severe toxemia]."

B_6 Solves Premenstrual Problems

There is hardly a woman who does not experience some discomfort before her period: tension, irritability, pain, acne flareups, weight gain, puffy hands and feet. How can B_6 help? At least two of these premenstrual problems, acne and swollen hands and feet, have yielded to a regimen of supplemental B_6.

ACNE. A skin specialist in Erie, Pennsylvania, B. Leonard Snider, M.D., gave daily B_6 supplements of 50 milligrams to 106 teenagers whose acne was under control, except for monthly flareups just prior to menstruation. In many cases the vitamin was taken for one week preceding and during the time of menstruation for an average of three menstrual periods. Seventy-six of the girls reported that B_6 reduced their acne anywhere from 50 to 75 percent (*Ob. Gyn. News,* May 1, 1974.)

WATER RETENTION. To find out what vitamin B_6 can do to reduce premenstrual water retention, let's return to the files of Dr. Ellis.

One evening, after finishing his hospital rounds, Dr. Ellis noticed a nurse with puffy hands and fingers. Intrigued, since he had recently been relieving the edema of pregnancy with B_6, he asked the nurse if her hands tingled or went to sleep—edema's most common symptoms.

"Dr. Ellis," the nurse replied, "there is something about this that has to do with my menstrual cycle. About midway between my periods is when I notice that the swelling and soreness begin. It lasts from seven to ten days and goes away when I menstruate."

Dr. Ellis's diagnosis: "premenstrual edema." And given his success in treating the edema of pregnancy with B_6, Dr. Ellis decided to pit the vitamin against this problem.

When the nurse came into his office the next day, Dr. Ellis prescribed two 50-milligram tablets of B_6 daily for five days, and asked her to return on the sixth day. She had this to report when she returned: "After taking the B_6 for two days my hands were better—in fact, seemed well. By the third day I was able to wear my rings, use the typewriter and sleep much better."

For the next 12 months, she took one 50-milligram tablet daily and had no pain or swelling. After a year, she took the tablets only on the ten days preceding menstruation and found equal relief.

Over the years, Dr. Ellis saw more and more patients with the same problem. In one group of women he treated for this disorder, 4 out of 11 had previously taken diuretics to control their puffiness with little success. But when they took 50 to 100 milligrams of B_6 daily, all their symptoms were relieved by the next cycle of menstruation.

New Hope for the Infertile

Women with unexplained infertility may find new hope for pregnancy in high doses of vitamin B_6, according to the findings of two gynecologists, Joel T. Hargrove, M.D., of Columbia, Tennessee, and Guy E. Abraham, M.D., of Rolling Hills, California. Twelve of 14 patients who had been infertile from 18 months to seven years were finally able to conceive after vitamin B_6 therapy. The study participants, ranging in age from 23 to 31, shared one thing in common—premenstrual tension.

Vitamin B_6 was given daily in doses ranging from 100 to 800 milligrams, depending on the dose needed to relieve each patient's tension symptoms. Of the 13 pregnancies that resulted (one woman conceived twice), 11 occurred within the first six months of therapy, one occurred in the seventh month and the last occurred in the eleventh month of the program. Although not sure why the patients became pregnant, Dr. Hargrove said there was a significant increase in levels of progesterone (a natural hormone which prepares the lining of the uterus to receive a fertilized egg) in five of seven women studied.

More Health Benefits from B₆

Those are the major benefits a woman gets from this all-important vitamin. But B_6 doesn't only liberate women from their health problems. A man or woman who has one or more of the following conditions may also benefit from extra B_6.

GALLSTONES DISSOLVE WITH B₆ AND CORN OIL. When the gallbladder is saturated with more cholesterol than it can handle, gallstones form. Once that happens, surgery is practically inevitable. But taken with corn oil, B_6 may provide a better and safer solution, according to Dr. K. Holub and his associates at the Wilhelmina Hospital in Vienna, Austria. In a carefully controlled study, 22 gallbladder patients were given one tablespoon of corn oil and two 25-milligram tablets of B_6 after gallbladder surgery. All patients were better able to keep their cholesterol under control, thereby reducing chances for future gallstone formation (*Acta Chirurgica Austriaca*, vol. 8, no. 4, 1976).

CONTROL OF KIDNEY STONES. Recurrent calcium oxalate stones are the most common kind of kidney stones plaguing people in the Western world. They represent about 70 percent of all kidney stones and may cause pain, fever, obstruction of the urinary passageway, infection and bloody urine.

Some researchers are finding B_6 an effective, convenient, inexpensive and harmless way to lower the rate of stone formation. Researchers in the Netherlands reported that one of their patients had had recurrent stone disease for 20 years. At the time of the study, she had been passing gravel daily. After being given high doses of vitamin B_6, her urinary oxalate was reduced to normal and no further stones were passed. She has continued taking B_6 and her condition has remained stable for 2 years, according to the report (*Kidney International,* September, 1979).

RELIEF FROM PAIN AND STIFFNESS. Another group that responds well to B_6 are people with pain, stiffness or swelling in the hands and fingers. Those problems are often the result of a neurological disease called the carpal tunnel syndrome, caused by the pressure of the wrist ligaments rubbing against the median nerve of the hand. Patients with this syndrome often complain of a burning or tingling sensation in the hands and fingers as well as morning pain and stiffness in the joints. They may also have a weak hand grip, and nighttime muscle spasms of brief paralysis.

Dr. Ellis has also pioneered B_6 therapy for carpal tunnel syndrome. In a study carried out jointly with Karl Folkers, Ph.D., and co-workers at the University of Texas Institute for Biomedical Research in Austin, Dr. Ellis treated ten people with severe pain and stiffness problems. Because all of these individuals were found to have a deficiency of B_6, the researchers decided to prescribe a relatively high dosage of the vitamin: 300 milligrams daily. The results were remarkable. Muscle spasms subsided. Swollen feet and ankles returned to normal so that larger shoe sizes could be abandoned. Knee pain and stiffness were eased so that patients could squat comfortably and get up and down better (*Research Communications in Chemical Pathology and Pharmacology,* April, 1976).

CONTACT LENS COMFORT. Conjunctivitis (inflammation of the inner surface of the eyelids and the outer surface of the eyes) has been helped with vitamin B_6. The vitamin therapy helped because it increased the flow of tears. Ned Paige, O.D., a Toronto, Canada, practitioner, realized that this approach might benefit patients whose inadequate tear flow made their contact lenses uncomfortable or unwearable. He used doses of 50, 100 and 500 milligrams daily. Responses at the lower levels were not especially satisfactory. However, in the group on 500 milligrams daily, six out of eight patients showed a significant response.

AUTISTIC CHILDREN RESPOND TO B$_6$. One of the most dramatic ways that large doses of B$_6$ have been used is to treat autistic children. These severely disturbed youngsters suffer from a stubborn psychosis that leaves them withdrawn and silent, virtually cut off from the outside world. But Bernard Rimland, Ph.D., director of the Institute for Child Behavior Research in San Diego, has seen amazing changes occur in these youngsters when given large amounts of B$_6$—usually several hundred milligrams—along with other nutrients, especially magnesium. Their behavior deteriorated noticeably when they stopped taking B$_6$ and rebounded just as sharply when they resumed. Without the vitamin, the children refused to talk. They would whine and shake nervously, hide under their blankets or retreat into their rooms. Interest and involvement in their surroundings shrank to a minimum. But with B$_6$, those same youngsters began to talk more, read, ask questions and play games. They became calmer and better able to socialize with their friends and family (*American Journal of Psychiatry*, April, 1978).

A Little Isn't Enough

Modern refining, processing, cooking and storage all deplete the reserves of B$_6$ in the food we eat, according to the late Henry A. Schroeder, M.D., an authority on trace nutrients. Summarizing laboratory analyses of hundreds of processed food products for their B$_6$ content in the May, 1971, issue of the *American Journal of Clinical Nutrition*, Dr. Schroeder said, "Large losses occurred as a result of the canning of vegetables, ranging from 57 to 77 percent. Frozen vegetables showed losses of 37 to 56 percent in the vitamin B$_6$." Frozen fruit juices, canned juices, canned meats and certain processed meats all lost B$_6$. About 80 percent of the B$_6$ is removed from wheat to make all-purpose flour. Precooked rice loses 93 percent of its original content of B$_6$.

That means the best bet for boosting our B$_6$ intake is to eat plenty of freshly cooked fish, lean meats and liver, plus sunflower seeds and filberts. (See table 5.) But if you have special needs for B$_6$—if you are a woman taking the Pill, have premenstrual pain and swelling, or have other B$_6$-related problems—you probably won't get as much of this nutrient as you need *even if you make a point of eating plenty of B$_6$-rich foods at every meal.*

Table 5
FOOD SOURCES OF VITAMIN B₆

Food	Portion	Vitamin B$_6$ (milligrams)
Banana	1 medium	0.89
Salmon	3 ounces	0.63
Mackerel, Atlantic	3 ounces	0.60
Chicken, light meat	3 ounces	0.51
Beef liver	3 ounces	0.47
Sunflower seeds	¼ cup	0.45
Halibut	3 ounces	0.39
Tuna, canned	3 ounces	0.36
Broccoli, raw	1 medium stalk	0.35
Lentils, dried	¼ cup	0.29
Brown rice, raw	¼ cup	0.28
Beef kidney	3 ounces	0.24
Brewer's yeast, debittered	1 tablespoon	0.20
Filberts	¼ cup	0.18
Buckwheat flour, dark	¼ cup	0.14

SOURCE: Adapted from
Pantothenic Acid, Vitamin B$_6$ and Vitamin B$_{12}$, Home Economics Research Report No. 36, by Martha Louise Orr (Washington D.C.: Agricultural Research Service, U.S. Department of Agriculture, 1969).

To get this vitamin in the amounts reported so beneficial by researchers, a daily supplement is absolutely essential, and for those with special needs, researchers are now advising anywhere from 10 to 100 times the Recommended Dietary Allowance of B$_6$. You have to be careful, though. Many multivitamin supplements still fail to deliver even the bare RDA of two milligrams daily.

If you don't have any of the health problems we've talked about, try taking a daily B complex supplement with, at the very least, two milligrams of B$_6$. Pregnant women, however, should have a daily B$_6$ intake of no less than ten milligrams. Be sure to look for a potency expressed in milligrams (mg.), not micrograms (mcg.). The former unit equals one-thousandth of a gram; the latter only one-millionth. And that's too little of a one-in-a-million vitamin like B$_6$.

Vitamin B₁₂ — More Than Anemia Protection

CHAPTER **6**

A superstar in the medical scene, B_{12} has had dramatic effects in the treatment of various nerve-related disorders—even in instances where conventional drugs and therapy have failed. But B_{12} is keeping you healthy even when it doesn't make the headlines. It's essential to normal cell production and growth, especially the formation and development of red blood cells. Those cells tote oxygen to every part of your body, and a lack of them—a disease called anemia—*weakens* every part of your body.

The Lifesaving Supplement

Scientists didn't always know about the link between B_{12} and anemia, though. The first hint of it came in 1934 when two physicians won the Nobel prize for discovering that patients with pernicious anemia (a specific and often deadly type of the disease) could be saved by eating large amounts of liver. A few years later, scientists realized that it was the high levels of B_{12} in the liver that countered the illness. Their finding spared some 10,000 lives each year in the United States alone!

And just look at the symptoms associated with this deadly disease. Fatigue. Weakness. Unsteadiness. Numbness and needle-and-pin sensations in the legs. Breathing difficulties. Weight loss. Loss of memory. Inflammation of the tongue. Abdominal discomfort. Chest pains. It's hard to believe that one vitamin can take care of all these symptoms. But when you consider that B_{12} plays an important role not only in red blood cell formation but also in the integrity of the central nervous system, then it's easy to understand what B_{12} means to our health and well-being. **31**

A Big Lift from B$_{12}$

That importance was underscored by an article in the scientific journal *Orthomolecular Psychiatry* (vol. 1, no. 1, 1972). H. L. Newbold, M.D., a New York City psychiatrist, described a case in which a 33-year-old patient came to him complaining of lethargy and depression. The young man was concerned because he was unable to complete work on his Ph.D. He had trouble dragging himself out of bed and to class in the morning. In class, he couldn't bring himself to participate in group discussions. And studying at home was becoming almost impossible since he found it difficult to comprehend or remember what he read.

Worst of all, he felt lonely, insecure and isolated. Two years before, he had had a nervous breakdown which resulted in marital problems. And since that time he had been subsisting on Thorazine, a powerful and commonly used drug in the treatment of psychiatric problems.

After running a series of laboratory tests, Dr. Newbold started the young man on injections of vitamin B$_{12}$. Two injections—and two weeks—later the patient returned markedly improved. He commented that his memory was much better and that he was learning well. In fact, for the first time in two years he was hard at work writing his Ph.D. thesis.

BACK FROM INSANITY. Dr. Newbold isn't the only one who believes that in certain cases B$_{12}$ may take the place of the psychiatrist's couch. Two Canadian physicians associated with McGill University and Jewish General Hospital in Montreal report dramatic results with B$_{12}$ in the treatment of a severely psychotic 35-year-old patient. Thorazine and even electroconvulsive (shock) therapy did not produce very encouraging results.

The next line of attack was nutritional. Nine years previously, the patient had undergone stomach surgery, a situation which frequently leads to a vitamin B$_{12}$ deficiency due to malabsorption. So the physicians tested for nutritional deficiencies. Surprisingly, his B$_{12}$ level fell in the "normal" range. But with no other game plan in mind they decided to give vitamin B$_{12}$ a try anyway.

The results were even better than anyone had hoped for. Eight days after B$_{12}$ therapy had begun the patient was released from the hospital with complete remission of his symptoms (*Diseases of the Nervous System*, vol. 36, no. 6, 1975).

MOCK SENILITY. In elderly people, B$_{12}$ deficiency can also set off a round of symptoms such as confusion, forgetfulness and depression that mimic senility—especially when low B$_{12}$ is coupled with a folate deficiency.

B$_{12}$ Shortage Reduces Fertility

Interestingly enough, B$_{12}$ has recently made headlines in an area which at first doesn't seem to have any relation to the central nervous system — fertility. Speaking recently at a conference on nutrition and reproduction held at the National Institutes of Health in Bethesda, Maryland, Jo Anne Brasel, M.D., noted that some women who cannot conceive — and for whom no medical reason can be found — may be deficient in vitamin B$_{12}$. Moreover, documented evidence has shown that conception leading to the birth of a normal infant may occur within a few short months of B$_{12}$ therapy.

And that bit of information is not for women only. "Furthermore," she added, "semen and sperm abnormalities have been noted in males with pernicious anemia. There is one spectacular case in which B$_{12}$ therapy led to return to active participation in sheep shearing by one 73-year-old Australian sheep herder — and pregnancy in his 37-year-old wife."

Making Sure You Get Your B$_{12}$

Animal foods are the only substantial dietary sources of vitamin B$_{12}$. Most doctors say that a B$_{12}$ deficiency is very rare; that with meat, milk and eggs being a mainstay of the American diet, it's assumed that we're taking in anywhere from 5 to 15 micrograms daily. (The Recommended Dietary Allowance for adults is 3 micrograms.)

But certain conditions may interfere with B$_{12}$ absorption, compromising health status. Various studies have shown that a number of drugs — including oral contraceptives — can lower blood concentrations of B$_{12}$. And physicians have long recognized that stomach or intestinal surgery often interferes with the body's production of stomach juices. In those stomach juices an "intrinsic factor" exists which combines with B$_{12}$ to aid in the vitamin's absorption. Without the intrinsic factor, a B$_{12}$ deficiency can develop despite a meaty diet.

Aging also causes changes in the gastrointestinal system which may lower the level of the intrinsic factors and cause poor absorption of B$_{12}$.

Also, many people who have been given vitamin B$_{12}$ tests and told that their B$_{12}$ levels were normal are actually suffering from a deficiency. It's been discovered recently that the B$_{12}$ test most commonly used — radiodilution assay — is highly unreliable. In fact, two physicians reporting in the *Journal of the American Medical Association* (October 24, 1980) call it "totally ineffective."

For those who have a serious deficiency of the vitamin —

particularly people who have gone years without proper treatment—B_{12} injections are preferred over oral supplementation. That way the vitamin bypasses the malabsorption problem in the stomach and goes directly to the depleted body tissues. However, in most cases, a dwindling intrinsic factor can be offset—and a low B_{12} level boosted back up to par—with a high dietary intake of B_{12}. Lean meat, poultry, fish, eggs and dairy products are good sources of the vitamin. (See table 6.) But by far the best source is beef liver.

Since B_{12} is found almost exclusively in animal foods, strict vegetarians—who shun meat, fish, eggs and dairy products altogether—run the risk of B_{12} deficiency. For that reason, vegetarians would be wise to include either a high-vitamin B_{12} yeast or B complex supplement in their daily diet.

But even if you eat plenty of meat and other animal foods, you may want to boost your B_{12} with supplements. If you've been ill, had surgery, or are getting on in years, diet alone probably won't be able to supply all your needs. Remember, sound nerves depend on it.

Table 6
FOOD SOURCES OF VITAMIN B$_{12}$

Food	Portion	Vitamin B$_{12}$ (Micrograms)
Beef liver	3 ounces	93.5
Lamb	3 ounces	2.6
Beef	3 ounces	2.0
Tuna, drained	3 ounces	1.8
Yogurt	1 cup	1.5
Haddock	3 ounces	1.4
Swiss cheese	2 ounces	1.0
Milk, whole	1 cup	0.9
Cottage cheese	½ cup	0.7
Egg	1 large	0.7
Cheddar cheese	2 ounces	0.4
Chicken, light meat	3 ounces	0.4

SOURCES: Adapted from
Pantothenic Acid, Vitamin B$_6$ and Vitamin B$_{12}$, Home Economics Research Report No. 36, by Martha Louise Orr (Washington, D.C.: Agricultural Research Service, U.S. Department of Agriculture, 1969).
Composition of Foods: Dairy and Egg Products, Agriculture Handbook No. 8-1, by Consumer and Food Economics Institute (Washington, D.C.: Agricultural Research Service, U.S. Department of Agriculture, 1976).

Folate, the Head-to-Toe Healer

CHAPTER 7

Folate (also known as folic acid or folacin) is another member of the B vitamin clan. Like all the other B vitamins, folate is critical to the functioning of the central nervous system. And being particularly concentrated in the spinal column—the hub of nervous system communications—folate might even be considered the big brother of the B vitamin family.

What happens when a folate deficiency interferes with that communication system? Static. In the body *and* the brain.

M. I. Botez, M.D., of the Clinical Research Institute of Montreal and Hotel-Dieu Hospital, Montreal, Canada, has described 16 cases which illustrate the varied physical and mental symptoms of a folate deficiency. According to Dr. Botez, a long list of disorders—including muscular weakness and cramping, physical and mental fatigue, forgetfulness, lack of concentration, insomnia, dizziness, depression, tension headaches, constipation and diarrhea—responded to folate treatment.

Motherhood Increases Folate Needs

A 29-year-old mother of two was written off as a hopeless hypochondriac, fraught with frazzled nerves, physical and mental fatigue, dizziness and tension headaches. Those troubles had all started after she gave birth to her second child, and were accompanied by muscle cramps, numbness and uncoordinated muscle movements in both arms and legs—all symptoms of a folate deficiency, according to Dr. Botez. Yet her physician had casually shrugged off these warning signs as psychosomatic in nature. Instead of folate supplements, he had prescribed tranquilizers and psychiatric counseling. Naturally, they didn't help.

35

Neurological examination upon admission to the hospital confirmed muscle weakness in the lower legs and depressed reflexes. A spinal tap was normal, but a blood test showed a low level of folate.

With folate therapy, her symptoms gradually lessened. And aside from a slight setback—when for three weeks her physicians substituted an inert substance just to test the actual effectiveness of folate—the young woman made steady improvement.

Eases "Restless Legs Syndrome"

One 76-year-old woman seen by Dr. Botez was extremely weak, particularly in her hands and feet. Her reflexes were slow and she had trouble coordinating her muscle movements. Besides that, she reported prickly, tingly sensations and burning in the soles of her feet.

Sound like a nervous system disorder? It was. Part of her problem—the numbness, weakness and pain in her legs and feet—is what doctors call the "restless legs syndrome." Interestingly enough, an editorial on the syndrome in the *Journal of the American Medical Association* (May 17, 1976) says that a physician "can offer little or nothing by way of treatment that the patient has not already found out for himself by experience." However, in Dr. Botez's study, the woman's restless legs syndrome was relieved when she was put on a regimen of folate.

Not only that, Dr. Botez reported marked improvement in her condition. Her reflex responses improved. Her ankles lost their spastic twitch. And her IQ even jumped with folate (*European Neurology*, vol. 16, no. 1-6, 1977).

Chase the Blues Away

Other Canadian physicians are looking into folate deficiency as a cause of depression. A study at McGill University, Montreal, examined the folate levels of three different groups of patients: those who were depressed, those who were psychiatrically ill but not depressed, and those who were medically ill. Six of the patients were men, 42 were women, and their ages ranged from 20 to 91.

The researchers discovered that "serum folic acid levels were signficantly lower in the depressed patients than in the psychiatric and medical patients. . . . On the basis of our results, we believe that folic acid deficiency depression may exist" (*Psychosomatics*, November, 1980).

Who Needs Folate?

Everybody. But some people have to be especially careful to get enough.

OLDER PEOPLE. According to a team of doctors at the New Jersey Medical School, people 70 or older are at greater risk of developing a folate deficiency, not so much because their folate intake is necessarily lower but because the aging body isn't capable of absorbing folate from food. To get around that problem, senior citizens should take folate as a supplement instead of relying on their diets, said Herman Baker, Ph.D., one of the researchers (*Journal of the American Geriatrics Society,* May, 1978).

"If an elderly person takes a good B complex vitamin which contains 100 micrograms of folate two times a day, he should satisfy his folate requirements," Dr. Baker told us. "The reason I stress a B complex supplement rather than a folate supplement is that it's very important for the person to be getting an adequate supply of vitamin B_{12}, as well. Otherwise, the folate might mask the symptoms of a B_{12} deficiency. And that could have serious consequences."

PREGNANT WOMEN. Eating for two means getting enough folate to compensate for the amount shunted to the growing fetus for development. Without an ample supply, both mother and child suffer. And for mom, that could mean a bout with postpartum depression, the so-called baby blues.

According to William E. Thornton, M.D., of the Medical University of South Carolina, one young woman who was unsuccessfully subjected to a whole host of tranquilizing drugs and even electroconvulsive (shock) therapy to ease her severe depression following childbirth responded well to folate therapy (*American Journal of Obstetrics and Gynecology,* September 15, 1977).

Nearly 50 percent of the ladies-in-waiting tested during one recent study were found to be lower in folate than nonpregnant women (*Journal of Nutritional Science and Vitaminology,* vol. 23, no. 5, 1977).

And with those low levels of folate, is it any wonder that the restless legs syndrome is so common among mothers-to-be? In a Canadian study, 21 pregnant women were given regular follow-ups during their pregnancies and six weeks after delivery, and at each visit they were rated for the severity of restless legs syndrome. Eleven of the women received a folate supplement, while the other 10 received a multivitamin that did not contain folate.

The results? Of the 9 women who had restless legs syndrome, only 1 had taken folate. However, of the 12 women who had no symptoms of restless legs, 10 had taken folate supplements. Said the researchers: "Our preliminary data suggest that restless legs syndrome in pregnancy could represent a sign of low serum folate concentration" (*Nutrition Reports International,* August, 1978).

During pregnancy, many women also suffer from inflamed gums—estimates range from as low as 30 to as high as 100 percent of them. A study of 30 women conducted during their fourth and eighth months of pregnancy showed that those who rinsed their mouths with a folate mouthwash twice daily for one minute experienced a "highly significant improvement" in the health of their gums during the eighth month (*Journal of Clinical Periodontology*, October, 1980).

WOMEN ON THE PILL might likewise do well to take a folate supplement. For some time, it's been noted that women who take birth control pills tend to have lower blood levels of various B vitamins, including folate. That may be due to increased losses, impaired absorption or redistribution to other tissues. In fact, it seems that much of the depression associated with women on the Pill comes from their depleted B vitamin stores. Makes sense.

Others at risk for folate deficiency are teenagers, nursing mothers, alcoholics, and people taking certain anticonvulsive, antibacterial or diuretic drugs.

Table 7
FOOD SOURCES OF FOLATE

Food	Portion	Folate (micrograms)
Brewer's yeast	1 tablespoon	313
Orange juice	1 cup	136
Beef liver	3 ounces	123
Black-eyed peas	½ cup	100
Romaine lettuce	1 cup	98
Beets	½ cup	67
Cantaloupe	¼ medium	41
Broccoli, cooked	½ cup	38
Brussels sprouts	4 sprouts	28

SOURCES: Adapted from
"Folacin in Selected Foods," by Betty P. Perloff and R. R. Butrum, *Journal of the American Dietetic Association*, vol. 70, February, 1977. *Nutritive Value of American Foods in Common Units*, Agriculture Handbook No. 456, by Catherine F. Adams (Washington, D.C.: Agricultural Research Service, U.S. Department of Agriculture, 1975).

Folate Foods Abound

As with many of the B vitamins, the best food sources of folate are organ meats such as liver, whole wheat products including wheat germ, and brewer's yeast.

Also, when you think folate, think foliage. The name folate is derived from the Latin word *folium,* or "leaf." And many green leafy vegetables (including broccoli, brussels sprouts and romaine lettuce) contain goodly amounts of folate. (Other foods with fairly large amounts of folate appear in table 7). But when you prepare those vegetables, just cook them as lightly as possible, because overcooking can destroy folate. Fresh cauliflower, for instance, cooked for as little as ten minutes in vigorously boiling water, loses 84 percent of its folate, reported Joseph Leichter, Ph.D., and

PABA, THE PROTECTIVE BONUS IN FOLATE

PABA (para-aminobenzoic acid) is considered a separate B vitamin by many nutritionists, but in fact it is a chemical component of folate. PABA occurs with the other B's in foods such as whole grains and brewer's yeast. Some evidence shows that PABA may help to lower blood fats and that it probably plays a role in maintaining the health of the female reproductive organs and in the normal uptake of the hormone estrogen. As a food supplement, PABA is available in tablet form.

But PABA is most widely recognized for its effective role in sunburn protection. When isolated and incorporated into suntan lotion, PABA screens out damaging UVB rays of the sun. UVB is the form of ultraviolet radiation that causes not only a painful and unsightly sunburn, but premature wrinkling and aging of the skin, and possibly precancerous changes. While blocking out those hazardous rays, PABA permits UVA rays—less dangerous, tanning rays—to seep through. You still tan, but more slowly and safely. Many people have already reported that taking PABA tablets by mouth helps protect them from the effects of the sun.

People with fair skin and blue or green eyes are the most susceptible to skin damage from the sun. But anyone who wants to enjoy the sunny outdoors without permanently ruining his or her skin should consider using PABA.

two co-workers at the University of British Columbia's Division of Human Nutrition in Vancouver, Canada. Other vegetables fared little better, with substantial portions of their folate content leaching into the cooking water (*Nutrition Reports International,* October, 1978).

So when you do cook, think about fast (but healthful) cooking methods for your vegetables, such as stir-frying.

The recommended allowance of folate for the normal adult is 400 micrograms per day. If you don't eat enough folate-rich foods, you may want to supplement your diet. If you're pregnant, the National Research Council advises you to make certain you're taking at least 800 micrograms of folate per day, and recommends 600 micrograms if you're nursing. Finally, if you're elderly, you may have trouble absorbing enough folate from the foods you're eating. Supplementation may be in order for you. (For more on supplements, see the chapter How Much Do You Need?)

Folate is a nutrient no one can afford to run short of. So whether you help yourself to seconds on vegetables or to a folate supplement, you'll be helping yourself immeasurably.

Pantothenate, the Antistress Vitamin

CHAPTER 8

Colitis. It's the disease God forgot to give Job. Even the "mild" variety comes complete with diarrhea and bloody stools. And severe colitis pulls out all the stops—literally. Diarrhea so constant the bathroom seems like a prison cell. Stomach cramps. Pale, feverish skin blotched with rashes. . . .

If this description is turning your stomach, please *don't* turn the page. We wanted to give you a really *dramatic* example of the role of pantothenate—one of the B complex vitamins. Perhaps the best way to see how a vitamin works to keep you healthy is to see how *un*healthy you can get when it's missing. And while colitis—a disease in which the colon is inflamed—is not caused by an outright deficiency of pantothenate, it may well be the result of the body's failure to efficiently utilize this vitamin.

Normally, your body uses pantothenate (also called pantothenic acid) by turning it into another substance, coenzyme A (CoA). Put another way, CoA is the metabolically *active* form of pantothenate. But researchers at the University of Manitoba, Winnipeg, Canada, and the Mayo Clinic in Rochester, Minnesota, found that although 29 patients with colitis had normal levels of pantothenate in their blood, the level of CoA in their colons was half of that found in the colons of 31 patients who did not have colitis (*American Journal of Clinical Nutrition,* December, 1976).

The researchers offered *six* possible explanations—all "speculations"—as to why colitis patients had low levels of CoA in their colons. Why the uncertainty? Because CoA is hard to pin **41** down. It helps the heart beat, the stomach digest, the lungs pump. And more.

Standing Up to Stress

CoA is vital in the health of your adrenal glands and in the production of the adrenal gland hormones, the hormones that give you the emotional and physical energy you need to cope with stress. *Any* stress. From a bitter argument to a bitter winter. From a traffic jam to jam spilled on your shirt. From a mosquito bite to the seven-year itch. In fact, CoA is so important for healthy adrenal glands that pantothenate (which turns into CoA) has been dubbed "the antistress vitamin."

Way back in the 30s, researchers had already discovered that rats deprived of pantothenate had severely damaged adrenal glands. They also found that rats fed a pantothenate-deficient diet reacted poorly to stress, while rats given extra pantothenate coped with stress better.

In one study, rats were divided into three groups. One group got a diet deficient in pantothenate. Another group got a diet adequate in pantothenate. The third group got a diet high in this vitamin. Then all the rats were put in cold water and made to swim until they were exhausted. The pantothenate-deficient rats swam an average of 16 minutes. The "adequate" group did better: They swam an average of 29 minutes. But the rats with a diet high in pantothenate swam an average of 62 minutes.

But what's true for rats is not necessarily true for us humans. So in 1952, Elaine Ralli and her co-worker, Mary Dumm, researchers in the department of medicine at the New York University-Bellevue Medical Center in New York City, tested the antistress effects of pantothenate on humans.

The researchers immersed a group of normal men in 48-degree water for eight minutes. Precise chemical measurements of the men's blood and urine were taken before and at intervals after the stress. Then, for six weeks, the men received ten grams of calcium pantothenate (a common form of pantothenate) every day. At the end of six weeks they were again immersed and the same measurements were taken.

Usually, stress causes a decrease in some of the white blood cells that protect the body against infection. After taking the pantothenate, the men had a "less pronounced" drop in these white blood cells. Also, levels of ascorbic acid (vitamin C)—a nutrient burned up by stress—were "significantly higher." And the men excreted less uric acid, a sign that the body had not undergone as much wear and tear. Importantly, they also had lower cholesterol levels (*Vitamins and Hormones*, vol. 11, 1953).

SPEEDS RECOVERY FROM SURGERY. A stress that's every bit as intense as cold water is the cold steel of a surgeon's knife. Fifty patients undergoing abdominal surgery were given 500 milligrams of panthenol—a substance similar to pantothenate—the day of surgery and for five days afterward. Another 50 patients were not given panthenol. The group receiving panthenol had quicker recoveries, with less nausea and vomiting—"a more benign postoperative course," in the words of the researchers conducting the study (*American Journal of Surgery*, January, 1959).

ARMOR AGAINST X-RAYS. But perhaps the most severe stress is x-ray radiation. Radiation is like tiny bullets shooting into the body and smashing cells to pieces.

In an experimental study, Dr. I. Szorady, of the department of pediatrics, University Medical School, Szeged, Hungary, exposed 200 laboratory mice divided equally into four groups to total body irradiation with x-rays. The rate of survival was highest in the group of mice receiving pantothenate for a week before irradiation. Half were still alive 21 days following the massive stress. But among 50 other mice *not* protected by supplemental pantothenate, half were dead within eight days of x-ray exposure (*Acta Paediatrica Hungaricae*, vol. IV, no. 1, 1963).

"It follows that, as compared to controls, survival was prolonged by 200 percent," Dr. Szorady concluded. "Due to its metabolic key position, pantothenic acid thus seems to induce slow biochemical processes which ensure enhanced protection against radiation injury."

These "slow biochemical processes" may be one key to how pantothenate shuts the door on stress.

Stress speeds you up. Thoughts flash through the mind. Blood pressure shoots up. The heart races. If you have a hard time steering through the stress in your life, your body may be in chronic fourth gear—but your health will come in last. Pantothenate may help keep your body moving at the speed it was built for.

A LONGER LIFE. Added proof for Dr. Szorady's theory of pantothenate's power to "slow biochemical processes" comes from Roger Williams, Ph.D., the first man to isolate, identify and synthesize pantothenate. Dr. Williams believes that pantothenate can actually prolong life. He conducted an experiment with two groups of mice, feeding both of them an identical and nutritionally complete diet. One group, however, got extra pantothenate in their drinking water.

The animals without extra pantothenate lived an average of 550 days. But those getting the extra pantothenate lived an average of 653 days.

"If the 550 days is regarded as equivalent to 75 years for a human, then the 653 days would be equivalent to 89 years," Dr. Williams wrote in *Nutrition Against Disease* (Pitman, 1971).

"On a purely statistical basis," he added, "I would be willing to wager that if a large number of weaned babies were given 25 milligrams of extra pantothenate daily during their lifetime, their life expectancy would be increased by at least ten years."

FEWER ALLERGIES. And they might have fewer runny noses, too. Dr. Szorady conducted a standard allergy skin test on 24 children, injecting them with the allergen histamine. "Pantothenic acid reduced the intensity of the skin reaction by 20 to 50 percent in all children," he reported. In his paper on pantothenate, he also cites a study in which a researcher "applied pantothenic acid treatment of allergic adults with satisfactory results."

RELIEVES BRUXISM. If you're in the habit of grinding your teeth—much to the annoyance of your spouse or roommate— pantothenate may help check the problem. According to Emanuel Cheraskin, M.D., D.M.D., and W. Marshall Ringsdorf Jr., D.M.D., bruxism (teeth grinding) is a nutritional problem that can be relieved with increased daily supplies of calcium and pantothenate. Drs. Ringsdorf and Cheraskin did a nutritional survey of a group of people, some of whom were bruxists. Those without bruxism recorded higher levels of pantothenate and calcium intake. A year later—after dietary instruction—the entire group was surveyed again. This time the doctors found that those bruxists who had significantly increased their intake of pantothenate and calcium were no longer tooth gnashers (*Dental Survey*, December, 1970).

There's more at stake here than an unpleasant habit. A Swiss dental scientist, Peter Schaerer of Bern, has said that people who clench their teeth during sleep or during a "confrontation" can cause damage to the teeth, gums, jaw joint and muscles (*Journal of the American Dental Association*, January, 1971).

Raw Foods a Must

You'd assume that nature would have stocked the pantry with a hefty supply of a vitamin so critical to overall health and well-being. And you'd be right. *Pantothen* is the Greek word for "from all sides," and pantothenate lives up to its name: It's found in almost all foods. But Mother Nature's pantry—brimming with vegetables, lean meats, whole grains, fruits, nuts and seeds—is a far cry from the pantry in most modern households where canned, frozen and highly processed foods crowd out the real thing. As far as pantothenate goes, these cupboards are just about bare.

That's because processed foods are losers. So concluded Henry A. Schroeder, M.D., author of a study entitled, "Losses of Vitamins and Trace Minerals Resulting from Processing and Preservation of Foods."

"It is apparent that raw foods supply adequate amounts [of pantothenic acid]...," wrote Dr. Schroeder. But, he continued, "It is not apparent, however, that persons subsisting on refined, processed and canned foods will be provided with adequate amounts...."

Facts back him up. When fresh vegetables are frozen, pantothenic acid gets the cold shoulder—the vegetables lose anywhere from 37 to 57 percent of this vitamin. Canned vegetables lose from 46 to 78 percent of their pantothenic acid. Processed and refined grains—the kind used in baking most of the breads, cakes, cookies, crackers and chips sold in supermarkets—lose 37 to 74 percent of this nutrient. Processed meats do no better, losing one-half to three-quarters (*American Journal of Clinical Nutrition,* May, 1971).

"These data," believed Dr. Schroeder, "cast doubt on the adequacy of the American diet for... pantothenic acid," and "demonstrate the dietary needs for the use of whole grains and unprocessed foods of most varieties."

And that goes double for babies. A recent Canadian study showed that processed, strained baby foods provide *only 25 percent* of an infant's need for pantothenate (*Nutrition Reports International,* June, 1977).

Another scientist who doubts whether most people get enough pantothenate is Dr. Klaus Pietrzik. Speaking to the 59th Annual Meeting of the Federation of the American Societies for Experimental Biology held in Atlantic City in April, 1975, Dr. Pietrzik warned that a diet with a 25 percent deficiency in pantothenic acid would damage the central nervous system after only six months. "The desirable doses of pantothenic acid possibly should be increased," he asserted. But what *are* the "desirable doses"?

It depends on whom you ask.

The No-Deficiency Diet

There is no Recommended Dietary Allowance for pantothenate. Why? "Insufficient evidence," according to the scientists responsible for setting the RDA. They believe, however, that "a daily intake of five to ten milligrams is *probably* [our emphasis] adequate for all adults," and "suggest" a ten-milligram intake for pregnant and lactating women.

Table 8
FOOD SOURCES OF PANTOTHENATE

Food	Portion	Pantothenate (milligrams)
Beef liver	3 ounces	4.8
Chicken liver	3 ounces	4.6
Beef kidney	3 ounces	2.6
Broccoli, raw	1 medium stalk	1.8
Beef heart	3 ounces	1.4
Turkey, dark meat	3 ounces	1.1
Brewer's yeast	1 tablespoon	1.0
Peanuts	¼ cup	1.0
Peas, dried	¼ cup	1.0
Chicken, dark meat	3 ounces	0.9
Egg, hard-cooked	1 large	0.9
Chicken, light meat	3 ounces	0.8
Milk, whole	1 cup	0.8
Mushrooms, raw	½ cup	0.8
Sweet corn	1 ear	0.8
Beef, lean	3 ounces	0.7
Sweet potatoes	1 medium	0.7
Cashews	¼ cup	0.6
Soybean flour	¼ cup	0.6
Turkey, light meat	3 ounces	0.6
Brown rice	¾ cup	0.5
Buckwheat flour, dark	¼ cup	0.4
Rye flour, dark	¼ cup	0.4
Whole wheat flour	¼ cup	0.3

SOURCES: Adapted from
Nutritive Value of American Foods in Common Units, Agriculture Handbook No. 456, by Catherine F. Adams (Washington, D.C.: Agricultural Research Service, U.S. Department of Agriculture, 1975).
Pantothenic Acid, Vitamin B_6 and Vitamin B_{12}, Home Economics Research Report No. 36, by Martha Louise Orr (Washington, D.C.: Agricultural Research Service, U.S. Department of Agriculture, 1969).
Composition of Foods: Poultry Products, Agriculture Handbook No. 8-5, by Consumer and Food Economics Institute (Washington, D.C.: Science and Education Administration, U.S. Department of Agriculture, 1979).
"Pantothenic Acid Content of 75 Processed and Cooked Foods," by Joan Howe Walsh, Bonita W. Wyse and R. Gaurth Hansen, *Journal of the American Dietetic Association,* February, 1981.
Composition of Foods: Dairy and Egg Products, Agriculture Handbook No. 8-1, by Consumer and Food Economics Institute (Washington, D.C.: Agricultural Research Service, U.S. Department of Agriculture, 1976).

That's one suggestion pregnant women should ignore, according to Dr. Williams. "I would be willing to give 10-to-1 odds that providing prospective human mothers with 50 milligrams of this vitamin per day would substantially decrease the number and severity of reproductive failures," he wrote in *Nutrition Against Disease.*

And while Dr. Szorady suggests a daily 15-milligram intake, he adds that "physical work, surgical intervention, injury, burns and grave infections, those of the gastrointestinal tract in particular, may double the pantothenic acid requirement of adults."

So how to meet your daily requirement?

Your best bet is not to fool with Mother Nature. Follow Dr. Schroeder's advice and include plenty of whole, unprocessed foods in your diet. Whole grains like brown rice, oats and whole wheat are good sources of pantothenate. A bowl of oatmeal sprinkled with wheat germ or bran is a good source. Eggs, too, supply plenty of pantothenate.

If you ask for dark meat at Thanksgiving, you'll have even more to be thankful for. The dark meat of turkey (and chicken) is an excellent source of pantothenate. Organ meats—especially liver—are also rich in the vitamin. B vitamin-packed brewer's yeast is another fine source of pantothenate. (See table 8.)

These foods, along with a B complex supplement with at least 10 milligrams of pantothenate, should supply you with more than enough of this vitamin. (Most B complex supplements have more than 10 milligrams of pantothenate; some have up to 100 milligrams. It may be listed as "pantothenic acid" or "calcium pantothenate" on the label.)

So if the stress in your life is getting you down, it's time you upped your intake of the antistress vitamin, pantothenate.

Biotin, Choline and Inositol, the Three Little B's

The last but not the least of the nutrients in the vitamin B complex health team are biotin, choline and inositol. Perhaps you've noticed them listed on the label of a bottle of vitamin supplements—and also noticed asterisks next to their names that lead your eye to a phrase like "Requirement in human nutrition not yet established." But that phrase doesn't mean that these three nutrients aren't important; it only means scientists have yet to discover *how much* of them you need to stay in good health.

On the Lookout for Biotin Deficiency

Most researchers and nutritionists have long believed that it is next to impossible to acquire a deficiency of biotin, because such small amounts are required (about 100 to 300 micrograms per day). What you don't pick up from the good food sources you eat (like liver, kidney, milk and eggs), said the scientists, the friendly bacteria that live in your large intestine will manufacture for you. (See table 9 for food sources of biotin.)

Between those two sources, how can anyone become deficient?

But apparently it's not that simple. "First of all," said Mary Marshall, research nutritionist with the U.S. Department of Agriculture's Human Nutrition Center, "many people have cut their intake of eggs and liver, the best sources of biotin, because of their high cholesterol content. I also think it's a myth that the bacteria in your gut can supply you with the biotin you're not getting in your diet. It's true that they make it, but they do it in the lower part of the large intestine, and absorption does not take

place at that location.

Table 9
FOOD SOURCES OF BIOTIN

Food	Portion	Biotin (micrograms)
Chicken liver	3 ounces	146
Calves' liver	3 ounces	45
Kidney, lamb	3 ounces	36
Oats, rolled, uncooked	½ cup	16
Egg, hard-cooked	1 large	12
Egg yolk	1 large	10
Haddock	3 ounces	5
Milk, whole or skim	1 cup	5
Halibut	3 ounces	4
Camembert cheese	2 ounces	3
Chicken, dark meat	3 ounces	3
Cod	3 ounces	3
Salmon	3 ounces	3
Tuna, canned in oil	3 ounces	3
Chicken, light meat	3 ounces	2
Lamb, shoulder, lean, raw	4 ounces	2
Orange	1 medium	2
Tomato, raw	1 medium	2
Turkey, dark meat	3 ounces	2
Whole wheat bread	1 slice	2
Black raspberries	½ cup	1
Cheddar cheese	2 ounces	1
Grapefruit	½ fruit	1

SOURCES: Adapted from
McCance and Widdowson's The Composition of Foods, by A.A. Paul and
D.A.T. Southgate (Elsevier/North-Holland Biomedical, 1978).
Nutritive Value of American Foods in Common Units, Agriculture
Handbook No. 456, by Catherine F. Adams (Washington, D.C.: Agricultural
Research Service, U.S. Department of Agriculture, 1975).
Composition of Foods: Dairy and Egg Products, Agricultural Handbook
No. 8-1, by Consumer and Food Economics Institute (Washington, D.C.:
Agricultural Research Service, U.S. Department of Agriculture, 1976).
Composition of Foods: Poultry Products, Agricultural Handbook No. 8-5,
by Consumer and Food Economics Institute (Washington, D.C.: Science
and Education Administration, U.S. Department of Agriculture, 1979).

"Besides," Mrs. Marshall told us, "we don't even know if we
have the same bacteria now as we did long ago, because of all the
antibiotics we've consumed over the years."

In fact, every time you take an antibiotic or sulfa drug, you may be killing off the biotin-manufacturing bacteria in your gut. So even if you could absorb the biotin they're making, they may not be there to make it.

ELDERLY AND ATHLETES BOTH NEED MORE. Even if you haven't taken an antibiotic in years, you still could be low in biotin, if you're physically active or elderly. A study done in Basle, Switzerland, measured the blood levels of biotin in various populations. The results showed that the elderly and athletes had significantly lower levels than the control group (*International Journal of Vitamin and Nutrition Research,* vol. 47, 1977).

"The elderly may have a problem with absorption," said Mrs. Marshall. "They do with many other nutrients, so it's possible that biotin is among them. We really don't know for sure."

"As for the athletes," speculated Herman Baker, Ph.D., an expert on biotin, "exercising causes a buildup of lactic acid in the muscles. Biotin is part of the enzyme system which is needed to break it down again. The more lactic acid that accumulates, the more biotin is needed."

HOSPITAL PATIENTS on total intravenous feeding should be aware that biotin deficiency can result. That's what happened recently to one little girl after three months on intravenous feedings. When she was given ten milligrams of biotin per day, she overcame the deficiency (*New England Journal of Medicine,* April 2, 1981).

BURNS AND SCALDS may call for a biotin boost, too. A study of nine children suffering from those injuries was conducted at the Institute of Child Health in London. Plasma biotin levels were significantly below the control values in all the children. "The evidence suggests," write the researchers, "that low plasma biotin levels found in children with burns and scalds are due to the injury either through loss of the vitamin or through increased requirements for tissue repair" (*Journal of Clinical Pathology,* vol. 29, 1976).

SUDDEN INFANT DEATH SYNDROME (SIDS) is a tragic phenomenon in which babies are found dead in their cribs for no apparent reason. It's been reported that SIDS is more common among bottle-fed babies than breastfed ones. That may be because a considerable loss of biotin occurs during the manufacture of certain infant formulas. It's been recommended that infant formulas be supplemented with biotin as a precaution against SIDS.

Choline Keeps Memories Sharp

Choline is a precursor or forerunner of acetylcholine, a brain compound that is essential for the smooth flow of nerve impulses. Studies have shown that extra choline in the diet increases levels of acetylcholine in the brain. Keeping all that in mind, it occurred to investigators at the National Institute of Mental Health that choline would aid memory. On two separate days they gave ten healthy volunteers, ranging in age from 21 to 29, either a supplement of ten grams of choline chloride or an identical-appearing but worthless substitute. Then after an hour and a half, the people were given two kinds of memory tests.

In the first, a serial learning test, subjects had to memorize in proper order a sequence of ten unrelated words. The list was read to each person and repeated as often as necessary until perfect recall was achieved and the list could be repeated twice in a row.

Choline significantly improved memory, reported research psychiatrist N. Sitaram, M.D., and his colleagues. In fact, people whose memories were the poorest improved the most. One individual who normally needed six trial readings to master the ten-word list cut that to four after taking choline. Another dropped from seven to five attempts with the choline supplement.

In the second test, the volunteers were read lists of 12 common words. Half the words were high-imagery, concrete words like "table" and "chair," which can be easily visualized. The rest were low-imagery words like "truth" and "late," which represent abstract, hard-to-visualize concepts and are more difficult to memorize.

In those trials, people didn't have to learn the lists in any particular order, but the words were read to them again and again until all 12 words could be successfully recalled twice in succession.

The results, as the authors describe them, were "extremely interesting." People didn't fare any better overall when they took choline, but when the second test was divided into high- and low-imagery words, they registered much better scores in the latter, more difficult category while taking the supplement. In other words, choline seemed to selectively enhance memory to meet the challenge of the tougher learning tasks (*Life Sciences,* vol. 22, no. 17, 1978).

That's quite encouraging. After all, who among us has never forgotten someone's name? Or returned from the supermarket without some of the items we intended to buy there? Or misplaced

Table 10
FOOD SOURCES OF CHOLINE

Food	Portion	Choline (milligrams)
Pure soybean lecithin	1 tablespoon	1,450
Beef liver	3 ounces	578
Egg	1 large	412
Fish	3 ounces	100
Soybeans, cooked	½ cup	36

SOURCE: U.S. Department of Agriculture Nutrient Data Research Group, 1981.

an important paper? And unlike certain drugs which also raise acetylcholine levels in the brain, the authors of that study point out that choline is a natural food component which is safe even in large amounts. The doses of choline given in these tests were at least ten times as great as the 900 milligrams or less supplied by a typical diet.

A NEW WEAPON AGAINST EPILEPSY? A doctor has theorized that choline may function as a natural anticonvulsant for people with complex partial seizure (CPS), a type of epilepsy, because when substances are present which interfere with choline's action, seizures increase. To test his theory, J. O. McNamara, M.D., associate professor of medicine at Duke University Medical Center in North Carolina, selected four patients with CPS whose drug therapy was not working. During the four-month study each patient was given choline along with his existing drug regimen. Doses started at 4 grams per day and were gradually increased to 12 or 16 grams per day by the third month. Blood levels of choline rose, seizures were briefer, and the patients felt less fatigue after the seizures.

"Choline therapy is probably not the be-all and end-all for epilepsy," Dr. McNamara told us, "but it does show promise."

Choline is found in lecithin, beef liver, eggs, fish and soybeans. (See table 10.)

Unexpected Benefits from Inositol

Inositol is synthesized in our body within individual cells. This substance appears in vital tissues and fluids such as the brain, heart and skeletal muscles, lungs, blood, mother's milk and liver. Inositol also shows up in a lot of nutritious foods. (See table 11.) And nature doesn't pack nutrients into foods just for practice. Flurries of research over the years point to bona fide value for dietary inositol.

LOWER FAT AND CHOLESTEROL. Back in the 1940s, a number of research teams found that inositol could bring about a noticeable reduction in blood levels of cholesterol. The ability of inositol to break up abnormal deposits of fat is dramatically seen in its use in the treatment of fatty infiltration of the liver. A study done with patients whose livers were uniformly infiltrated with fat as a complication of gastrointestinal cancer showed that administration of inositol and choline reduced liver fat to normal levels in less than 24 hours (*Proceedings of the Society for Experimental Biology and Medicine,* vol. 54, 1943, abstract no. 14345).

HELP FOR MS. A Danish researcher believes that multiple sclerosis may be caused by an intermittent deficiency of the B vitamin inositol. Viggo Holm, M.D., writes in the July, 1978, issue of *Archivos de Neurobiologica* that in people with multiple sclerosis, the body's metabolism of inositol may be abnormally rapid. That would result in a deficiency of inositol, which would lead to the destruction of the myelin sheaths protecting and insulating the nerves.

Dr. Holm tested the metabolism of 86 normal people and 12 people with multiple sclerosis and found that none of the normal people metabolized inositol abnormally. However, 27 percent of the MS patients did metabolize inositol "in an abnormally pronounced way."

DIABETICS CAN BENEFIT. In treating diabetes today, doctors are paying closer attention to vitamins and minerals. Deficiencies of vitamins B_6 and B_2 are not uncommon among diabetics, studies have shown, and often complicate the disease. Now it seems that a form of inositol known as myoinositol may be involved in preventing the nerve damage that often causes pain, numbness and impotence in diabetics. After clinical trials with 15 patients, Rex S. Clements, M.D., associate director for clinical programs at Diabetes Hospital, Birmingham, Alabama, reports "a statistically significant improvement in nerve function on the high-myoinositol diet."

Sources of inositol are easy to find—particularly among high-fiber, high-carbohydrate natural foods. They include cantaloupes, citrus fruits, peanuts and whole grains. (See table 11.)

So when you think of B vitamins, don't forget the three little B's. They could help you out in a big way.

Table 11
FOOD SOURCES OF INOSITOL

Food	Portion	Inositol (milligrams)
Grapefruit juice, made from frozen concentrate	1 cup	912
Orange juice, made from frozen concentrate	1 cup	490
Great Northern beans	½ cup	440
Cantaloupe	¼ medium	355
Orange	1 medium	307
Wheat bread, stone ground	1 slice	288
Kidney beans	½ cup	249
Navy beans, dried	¼ cup	142
Peanut butter, creamy	2 tablespoons	122
Chicken liver	3 ounces	118
Green beans	½ cup	105
Almonds	¼ cup	99
Potato, baked	1 medium	97
Oatmeal, cooked	1 cup	84
Split peas	½ cup	65
Beef liver	3 ounces	58
Green pepper, cooked	½ cup	57
Tomato, raw	½ cup	54
Zucchini	½ cup	53
Pork chop	3 ounces	38
Onions, raw	¼ cup	22

SOURCE: Adapted from
"Myo-inositol Content of Common Foods: Development of a High-myo-inositol Diet," by Rex S. Clements Jr., and Betty Darnell, *American Journal of Clinical Nutrition,* September, 1980.

Vitamin C for Common and Uncommon Ailments

In 1747, James Lind proved that lemon juice could prevent scurvy, the disease that ravaged sailors on long voyages. Years later, scientists realized it was the *vitamin C* in lemon juice that cured the disease, which was the most severe stage of a vitamin C deficiency. But in the 20th century, scientists have discovered that vitamin C (also known as ascorbic acid) can do a lot more than keep people from getting scurvy. Among modern sailors on a Polaris submarine, for instance, 37 crew members who took 2,000 milligrams of vitamin C a day had 66 percent fewer cold symptoms than sailors who took a placebo, a fake pill (*International Research Communication System,* May, 1973).

Super Health with Super C

And when it comes to dealing with colds and other ills of the respiratory tract, vitamin C may do a lot more than just ease the problem. Sometimes it solves it.

COLDS, ASTHMA AND ALLERGIES. Study after study shows that people who take vitamin C have fewer and milder colds. At the University of Toronto, Canada, 407 people received 1,000 milligrams of vitamin C a day and an extra 3,000 milligrams a day for the first three days of a cold. Another 411 people received a placebo. Compared to the placebo group, the people who took vitamin C spent 30 percent fewer days indoors because of illness and missed 33 percent fewer days of work (*Canadian Medical Association Journal,* September 23, 1972). **55**

In a study of soldiers undergoing training in northern Canada, those receiving 1,000 milligrams of vitamin C a day had about 68 percent less illness than a placebo group (*Report No. 74–R–1012,* Defense Research Board, Department of National Defense, Canada, 1974).

And in another study from Toronto, 448 people who took vitamin C had up to 38 percent fewer cold symptoms—runny nose, fever, sore throat, tight chest, aching limbs, depression—than a placebo group.

"There is little doubt," wrote the authors of the Toronto study, "that the intake of additional vitamin C can lead to a reduced burden of winter illness" (*Canadian Medical Association Journal,* April 5, 1975).

Other studies have shown that vitamin C is effective in relieving asthma attacks. One of the most recent studies was conducted by two scientists at Yale University. It concentrated on vitamin C's ability to relieve exercise-induced bronchospasm in asthmatics.

"All asthmatics have this syndrome to some extent, and in a number of asthmatics it's the prominent feature of their disease," said E. Neil Schachter, M.D., one of the researchers involved. "Characteristically what happens is that an asthmatic will engage in a sport, or some kind of exercise, and feel fine throughout the activity. But then 3 to 5 minutes after the exercise, he'll feel a tightness in his chest and will start wheezing. The attack tends to get progressively worse over the next 30 minutes."

Patients in the study at Yale were pretreated with 500 milligrams of vitamin C before an exercise test. The vitamin C significantly lessened the severity of the bronchospasm following the exercise (*Chest,* September, 1980).

Dr. Schachter told us that vitamin C is by no means the most effective agent for reducing bronchospasm, but that it does have other advantages. "The problem with drugs which traditionally have been used with asthmatics is that they produce undesirable side effects—things like nervousness, upset stomach, or worse. Vitamin C has the potential to help asthmatics, with a lot less of these unpleasant or dangerous side effects."

Allergies, too, may be helped by vitamin C. The symptoms of nasal allergy—runny nose, inflamed and swollen mucous membranes—are caused by histamine, a chemical in the body. Vitamin C, studies show, is a natural *anti*histamine.

Researchers had 17 healthy volunteers inhale histamine and measured their levels of "airway constriction." The next day, the volunteers again received histamine—but this time they got 500 milligrams of vitamin C first. With vitamin C, the degree of airway constriction was "significantly smaller" (*Journal of Allergy and Clinical Immunology*, April, 1973).

For more on nutrition and colds, see the chapter on vitamin A.

PERIODONTAL (GUM) DISEASE, also known as pyorrhea, is an insidious deterioration of the gums and underlying jawbone marked by inflammation and infection. Periodontal disease is the main reason teeth loosen and fall out as we age. The cause is thought to be an invisible buildup of plaque—food debris, dead cells and bacteria—that coats our teeth at the gum line.

But a mild vitamin C deficiency may be another cause of pyorrhea, claims Olav Alvares, D.D.S., Ph.D., an associate professor of oral biology at the University of Washington in Seattle. Dr. Alvares told us that slightly lower than normal levels of vitamin C in the blood—a common problem—may spark the development of inflamed and bleeding gums. To study the connection between vitamin C deficiency and susceptibility to periodontal disease, the investigator used two groups of monkeys. Four animals were fed a nutritionally adequate diet and vitamin C supplements. Six other experimental monkeys received diets deficient in vitamin C and no extra nutrient boosts.

After researchers induced periodontal disease during the study's 23rd week, Dr. Alvares noted a "greater inflammatory response" in the vitamin C-deficient group. He believes the animals' "susceptibility to periodontitis" may be related to a poor showing by their white blood cells, bacteria-eating cells which need vitamin C to function.

URINARY TRACT INFECTIONS, or UTI, are the most uncomfortable kind of infections going. Millions of people—mostly women—get bladder infections (cystitis) every year. UTI can also affect other parts of the urinary system—the urethra (the tube that vents urine from the bladder) or the kidney itself. The infections are caused by any number of treacherous bacteria, but most often by *E. coli*.

Vitamin C can stop those bacteria in their tracks. "Its presence in the urine may actually promote good health in the bladder and kidneys," said Alan Gaby, M.D., of Kent, Washington. "Vitamin C can kill some bacteria, including *E. coli,* the most common cause of urinary tract infections. That killing power is especially strong at the uniquely high vitamin C levels that are possible in the concentrated fluid of urine. Doctors have used vitamin C for years to prevent urine infections in people likely to develop them. It's generally assumed that the vitamin works by producing an acid urine which inhibits the growth of bacteria. In fact, vitamin C does a poor job of acidifying the urine. The effectiveness of the vitamin is more likely related to a direct bactericidal [bacteria-killing] action."

Beyond Immunity

It's clear that vitamin C is a cornerstone of immunity. But there's more to tip-top health than squelching sneaky germs. From sudden accidents to long-standing health problems, vitamin C can come to the rescue.

WOUND HEALING. Vitamin C tops the list of wound-healing vitamins. Whether you've been cut, punctured, broken, bruised or burned, vitamin C is essential for the most important part of the healing process—the formation of collagen, the glue which puts and holds cells together. Anybody deficient in vitamin C may not be able to form collagen, and that means wound healing may be delayed or might never take place. For example, when patients with persistent bedsores were given supplements of two 500-milligram tablets of vitamin C a day, they healed twice as fast (*Lancet,* September 7, 1974). And in another study, investigators found that, in over a thousand patients, wound infections worsened when blood levels of ascorbic acid fell (*Journal of the Indian Medical Association,* February, 1975).

For more about nutrition and wound healing, see the chapter on vitamin E.

HEART DISEASE. A study in India found that when patients with a history of heart disease were given two grams of C a day, there were significant changes in several important components of their blood. Cholesterol levels dropped 12 percent, low-density lipoproteins (LDL) were down significantly and high-density lipoproteins (HDL) were up. The lipoproteins are complexes of fat and protein in the blood. Low-density lipoproteins appear to increase the risk of heart disease, while high-density lipoproteins protect against it, so C moved *all* the important indicators in a healthy direction.

Vitamin C may also have changed the tendency of the patients' blood to form clots. Heart attacks take place when blood clots close off the supply lines of nutrients and oxygen to the heart muscle. The inclination of particles in the blood called platelets to stick together contributes to the formation of blood clots, and patients receiving two grams of C daily were found to have less adhesive platelets.

Also, when a person's blood clots, an insoluble protein called fibrin is formed. In patients with a past history of heart disease, vitamin C increased the destruction of fibrin by 45 percent. In tests with patients currently suffering from heart disease, the figures were even more dramatic, with the destruction of fibrin up 62.5 percent. That anticlotting action could mean greater protection against heart disease.

The findings are particularly impressive when you consider that none of the people in the Indian study were deficient in vitamin C, at least according to the standard definitions of vitamin deficiency. The supplements given the patients made a difference even though all were supposedly already getting all the C they needed (*Atherosclerosis,* vol. 35, no. 2, 1980).

More recently, a study in England showed that 11 elderly hospital patients with coronary artery problems who took one gram (1,000 milligrams) of vitamin C daily had a decrease of total blood cholesterol levels in only six weeks. What's more, that benefit was not restricted to the heart patients; 7 healthy people given vitamin C also had lower cholesterol.

As a result of the study, the research team has entered a plea for a higher recommended daily intake of vitamin C because "latent ascorbic acid deficiency may be one of several preventable 'risk' factors contributing to the present epidemic of heart disease in the Western world" (*Journal of Human Nutrition,* vol. 35, no. 1, 1981).

For more on nutrition and heart disease, see the chapter on vitamin E.

CANCER. Other researchers have been closely examining vitamin C's effects on cancer cells. In a study at the University of Kansas Medical Center, researchers recently found that vitamin C suppressed the growth of certain leukemia cells. The scientists took bone marrow cells from 28 leukemia patients and placed them in 28 special containers (cultures). In 7 of the 28 cultures, the numbers of leukemic cell colonies were reduced markedly when vitamin C was added (*Cancer Research,* April, 1980).

A group of researchers from France and Texas found that vitamin C stops the growth of another type of cancerous cell—a melanoma. In their study, the researchers extracted both cancerous and noncancerous cells from mice. Then they placed the cells in two separate cultures and added vitamin C. The cancerous melanotic cells showed a 50 percent decrease in colony formation, cell number and their ability to stay alive.

"Vitamin C may directly inhibit the growth of proliferating cells, and this might explain some of the reported carcinostatic [cancer-suppressing] effects," the researchers write (*Nature,* April, 1980).

Most of those "effects" have been reported by Linus Pauling, Ph.D.—better known, perhaps, for his enthusiasm for the power of vitamin C to prevent the common cold. Along with Ewan Cameron, a Scottish surgeon, Dr. Pauling has reported that daily supplements of vitamin C in large amounts can add many precious days—and sometimes years—to the lives of "terminal" cancer patients (patients who are not expected to live).

In one of their clinical studies, Drs. Cameron and Pauling compared the survival time of 100 terminal cancer patients selected over a five-year period and given vitamin C, with 1,000 similar patients who did not receive the vitamin. Each person receiving vitamin C was matched with 10 "control" patients of the same sex, close to the same age, and suffering from the same type of tumor, who did not get vitamin C.

People receiving vitamin C started out with ten grams (10,000 milligrams) a day intravenously. That was usually stopped after about ten days, and then the patients began to take the same dosage by mouth.

In every type of cancer treated, the people receiving vitamin C tended to live longer—up to four times longer—than those who did not receive the vitamin. Lung cancer patients, for example, survived an average of 3.53 times longer after being declared untreatable than did their controls. Those with stomach cancer lived 2.61 times longer. Bladder cancer victims survived 4.49 times longer. Patients with kidney tumors displayed a greater than fivefold increase in life expectancy. Those with breast cancer lived 5.75 times longer. And those with cancer of the colon managed to survive on the average 7.61 times longer on the vitamin C regimen.

What's more, many of the people receiving vitamin C reported less pain. They were able to get by with less dependence on painkilling drugs. In short, they not only lived longer, they found life more worthwhile (*Proceedings of the National Academy of Sciences,* October, 1976).

PRICKLY HEAT. The intense burning and itching sensation of prickly heat is caused by a blockage of the sweat ducts. Strained by intense heat and humidity, the body's evaporative cooling system breaks down. Instead of being exuded through the pores, sweat becomes trapped beneath the skin, and results in a rash that feels like its name. But, according to a study carried out in Singapore by dermatologist T. C. Hindson, prickly heat is no match for vitamin C.

Dr. Hindson studied 30 children who had been plagued continuously by prickly heat for at least eight weeks prior to the test. Half the youngsters were given a placebo and the other half vitamin C.

After two weeks, the rash had disappeared completely on 10 of the 15 children receiving vitamin C. Four others showed improvement and 1 remained unchanged. By contrast, 9 youngsters in the placebo group showed no change and 2 had gotten worse. The rash had either cleared up or improved in the other 4.

The 11 children in the placebo group whose prickly heat had either shown no improvement or actually worsened were then given vitamin C and checked after two more weeks. The rash had cleared completely in 6 children and improved in the other 5.

Admitting that the exact mechanism at work remained unclear, Dr. Hindson concluded that vitamin C, when given in high doses, is "effective in the treatment and prevention of prickly heat." He also noted one of the vitamin's greatest advantages: "No unwanted side effects have been recorded from such doses to date" (*Lancet*, June 22, 1968).

Your Personal Defense against Pollution

Vitamin C has been reported to interact with over 50 chemical pollutants, modifying the dangers of arsenic, cadmium, cyanide, lead, mercury, benzene, vinyl chloride, carbon monoxide, ozone, PCBs and several insecticides. We'll highlight just a few of the specific environmental insults against which vitamin C protects us.

OZONE is one of the air pollutants that make up smog's chemical soup. When scientists tested the loss of vitamin C from the lung tissue of mice exposed to ozone, they found that as much as 50 percent of the vitamin in the lungs was lost when the mice breathed the chemical. But scientists also have established that extra vitamin C in the diet can *prevent* lung damage caused by breathing ozone (*Chemico-Biological Interactions*, vol. 30, no. 1, 1980). See the chapter on vitamin E for more on nutritional steps against pollution.

SMOKING robs you of vitamin C. Pack-a-day puffers had 25 percent less vitamin C in their blood than nonsmokers, a Canadian survey discovered. And those who smoked more than a pack a day faced a 40 percent deficit.

Some scientists think that smokers have such low levels of vitamin C because their bodies use up the nutrient to detoxify cadmium, a substance in cigarette smoke—and, unfortunately, a pollutant in food, water and air. So even nonsmokers may need extra vitamin C to fight cadmium.

NITRITES AND NITRATES are chemical substances added to cured meats, bacon and hot dogs as preservative and coloring agents. The trouble starts, however, when these two chemicals react with other substances. Nitrate reacts easily in nature to form the more dangerous nitrite, and nitrite reacts with chemicals called amines and amides to produce nitrosamines and nitrosamides, highly potent cancer causers. Nitrosamines and nitrosamides can form in liquor, in cured meats and fish and in cigarette smoke.

There is a growing body of evidence that vitamin C blocks the formation of nitrosamines and nitrosamides. In 1972, a team of scientists headed by Sidney Mirvish, Ph.D., working at the Eppley Institute for Research in Cancer in Omaha, Nebraska, found that vitamin C successfully competes with amines for the nitrite, using it up and preventing the formation of nitrosamines. Dr. Mirvish suggested that those drugs and foods containing nitrite be combined with vitamin C to prevent the formation of nitrosamines in the stomach (*Science,* July 7, 1972).

That suggestion is crucial, because vitamin C and nitrites must be in the stomach *at the same time* to prevent the harmful transformations that can lead to cancer, according to John Weisburger, Ph.D., who's studied nitrosamines. "Food stays in the stomach for two or three hours. So drinking a glass of orange juice at seven o'clock and eating nitrite-treated foods at eight may work, but the two shouldn't be ingested too far apart," Dr. Weisburger told us. "Vitamin C should either be added to the food or be a part of the meal."

PCBs (POLYCHLORINATED BIPHENYLS) are unique chemicals formulated in 1927 that resist destruction even by super-high temperatures or corrosive acids. Chemicals that can persist in the environment for decades—and have. They are *the* most widespread chemical pollutants, found everywhere from the polar ice caps to 11,000 feet under the ocean. And chemicals that, even in extremely low doses, can cause ill health—severe acne, cysts, skin discoloration, abdominal pain, nausea and loss of appetite, impotence, bloody urine and fatigue. Long-term exposure produces infertility.

Over 90 percent of all Americans have detectable levels of PCBs stored in their fatty tissues, levels often as high as 10 parts per million (ppm). And Lester Crawford, Ph.D., an FDA official, told us that the problem is getting worse.

"Since there is a low-level exposure to PCBs all the time and since the chemicals accumulate in the body, body levels of PCBs will go up in the future. I would project a level of 50 ppm in human tissue. That shouldn't cause acute illness. But," Dr. Crawford warned, *"it may have a lot of chronic effects we don't even know about yet."*

Rather than wait around for years—even decades—before government and industry figure out how to guard us from PCBs, you'd be better off protecting yourself now. Vitamin C may help shield us against PCBs.

In a study of vitamin C and PCBs, researchers fed young experimental animals high doses of the chemical. The animals grew poorly and had high levels of cholesterol. (PCBs are known to interfere with fat metabolism.) The animals also excreted 44 *times* more vitamin C in their urine—a sign, said the researchers, that the animals' bodies were synthesizing large quantities of the vitamin in an attempt to detoxify PCBs.

Next the researchers fed another group of experimental animals PCBs—but also gave them vitamin C. These animals grew normally and had normal cholesterol levels. They also had a "normal outward appearance," compared to the sickly appearance of the PCB animals who didn't get vitamin C (*Nutritional Reports International,* February, 1977).

Reach for the C

Table 12 shows some of the very best food sources of vitamin C. Because vitamin C is heat- and water-soluble, foods supplying this nutrient should be cooked as lightly as possible. A potato boiled in its skin, for instance, loses only 20 percent of its vitamin C while hashed brown potatoes, on the other hand, part with 70 percent of their vitamin C during cooking.

The Recommended Dietary Allowance for vitamin C is 60 milligrams a day for an adult—a little more than enough to prevent scurvy. Dr. Linus Pauling believes in taking ten grams (10,000 milligrams) a day of vitamin C to beef up immunity. The answer to just how much you as an individual may need lies somewhere in between. Sixty milligrams of vitamin C will no doubt keep you from getting scurvy—spongy, bleeding gums and overall weakness—but more is probably necessary to speed healing, combat pollution, lower cholesterol, and so on. (To help you determine your individual needs for vitamin C, see the chapter How Much Do You Need?)

For optimum effectiveness, vitamin C should be taken in divided doses throughout the day, rather than in one large amount. That's because excess vitamin C—more than the body can promptly absorb—is dumped into the urine. Divided doses provide a more evenly distributed supply of C, enabling the body to use as much as possible.

And that, hopefully, will enable you to stay as healthy as possible.

Table 12
FOOD SOURCES OF VITAMIN C

Food	Portion	Vitamin C (milligrams)
Orange juice, fresh-squeezed	1 cup	124
Green peppers, raw, chopped	½ cup	96
Grapefruit juice	1 cup	93
Papaya	½ fruit	85
Brussels sprouts	4 sprouts	73
Broccoli, raw, chopped	½ cup	70
Orange	1 medium	66
Turnip greens, cooked	½ cup	50
Cantaloupe	¼ medium	45
Cauliflower, raw, chopped	½ cup	45
Strawberries	½ cup	44
Tomato juice	1 cup	39
Grapefruit	½ fruit	37
Potato, baked	1 medium	31
Tomato, raw	1 medium	28
Cabbage, raw, chopped	½ cup	21
Blackberries	½ cup	15
Spinach, raw, chopped	½ cup	14
Blueberries	½ cup	10
Cherries, sweet	½ cup	8
Mung bean sprouts	¼ cup	5

SOURCE: Adapted from
Nutritive Value of American Foods in Common Units, Agriculture Handbook No. 456, by Catherine F. Adams (Washington, D.C.: Agricultural Research Service, U.S. Department of Agriculture, 1975).

Strong Bones Rely on Vitamin D

CHAPTER 11

A disease caused by darkness. A disease of buckling spines, of back pain and fatigue. A disease that zeroes in on the elderly—particularly elderly women. A disease most doctors fail to diagnose. But a disease you can prevent—or cure—with exercise, adequate calcium and phosphorus, and a very important nutrient: vitamin D.

The disease, osteomalacia, is a bone disorder in which the skeleton becomes demineralized. Bone is not a static chunk of minerals, but living tissue whose cells undergo a complete turnover every four months. Normally, new bone is as strong as old bone. But in osteomalacia, new bone is soft—it lacks the mineral calcium. *The lack is caused by a deficiency of vitamin D,* a nutrient which allows the absorption of calcium through the intestines into the bones.

Sunshine's Gift to Healthy Bones

Vitamin D deficiency, however, is not so much a *dietary* deficiency as a *sunlight* deficiency. Sunlight turns a chemical in your skin into vitamin D. Until winter comes. Then your skin is in virtual darkness—the short days and long nights leave you little time to spend outdoors, and during those few moments you bundle up in clothes. Month by winter month, vitamin D levels fall—until, perhaps, your bones begin to fall apart.

To find out *exactly* how low vitamin D drops in winter, researchers in England chose 23 older people and measured their blood levels of vitamin D every 3 months for 16 months (*British Medical Journal,* August 4, 1979). Taking the first measurement in **65**

July, 1975, they found the group had normal levels of vitamin D. By November of that year, however, the levels had dropped by an average of 19 percent. By February of 1976, they had dropped 65 *percent*—to a point where 9 of the group had levels "within the range that osteomalacia may be expected to develop." The May measurement showed a slight increase, but it was still 62 percent below the previous summer. July of 1976 found the levels back to normal—but by October they had begun to drop again.

DIET ALSO LOW IN D. The levels were low in winter not only because of a lack of sunshine, said the researchers, but because "dietary vitamin D intakes are inadequate." The researchers found that the amount of vitamin D in the group's diet—mainly from vitamin D-fortified dairy products, fish and eggs—"was generally too low to make a biologically important contribution to maintaining vitamin D concentrations."

The 23 people, they discovered, had an average daily vitamin D intake of 96 I.U.—but the researchers believe more than 200 I.U. a day may be needed to prevent osteomalacia.

POLLUTION ADDS TO THE PROBLEM. Yet the bleak sunshine of winter *and* low dietary levels of vitamin D are not the only causes of vitamin D deficiency. Day after day, winter and summer, the amount of vitamin D that sunlight forms in your body is being slowly reduced—by pollution.

Increased ozone from car exhaust and industry cuts down the amount of ultraviolet light (UVL) reaching the earth. (UVL is the part of sunlight that sparks the formation of vitamin D.) The amount of ozone in the air has steadily increased over the past few decades, and a group of researchers estimates "that in the period from 1951 to 1972 the total vitamin D accumulation by the body might have thus been reduced by 15 percent.

"It might be expected," they continue, "that the 15 percent decrease in total vitamin D accumulation . . . might be reflected by an increase in . . . osteomalacia in the elderly population" (*Aviation, Space and Environmental Medicine,* June, 1976).

To support their theory, the researchers cite two studies conducted in the 1970s in which approximately 40 percent of women who had broken a hip were found to have osteomalacia.

Bones Don't Break

But *whatever* decreases vitamin D levels—winter, poor diet or pollution—increases the chances of breaking your hip, according to some British researchers. They compared the blood vitamin D levels of two groups: 98 women 65 and over who had been hospitalized for a hip fracture and 76 similar women who had not broken a hip. *The average vitamin D level of the fracture group was 38 percent lower than that of the healthy group.* The researchers also found that the fracture group had an average daily intake of vitamin D that was 21 I.U. lower than that of the healthy group, with 58 percent of the fracture group getting less than 100 I.U. a day compared to 41 percent of the healthy group (*British Medical Journal,* March 3, 1979).

But those women could have increased their vitamin levels and perhaps prevented their hip fractures by taking vitamin D. Researchers gave 500 I.U. of vitamin D a day to older people who had low blood levels of the nutrient. "By two months," the researchers write, "vitamin D produced a significant increase" in blood vitamin D levels. In one group, levels rose over 500 percent from August, when they began taking the supplements, to February of the following year—at which point their levels were almost the same as those of "healthy young adults" (*British Medical Journal,* October 1, 1977).

In light of that success, the researchers strongly recommend that older people take a vitamin D supplement: "A dose of 500 I.U. vitamin D daily should therefore produce adequate blood [vitamin D] concentrations in most old people, and probably prevent most cases of osteomalacia in the elderly."

If 500 I.U. of vitamin D is good, is more better? No. The researchers gave some groups 2,000 I.U. a day of vitamin D. After six months, the vitamin D levels in those groups were "only marginally higher than those in subjects on 500 I.U."

But osteomalacia is not the most common bone disease. Osteoporosis is—a disease one doctor calls "the greatest epidemic among the elderly."

Osteomalacia is a disease of *quality*—the bone lacks calcium. Osteoporosis is a disease of *quantity*—the bone is normal, but there is less of it. In osteoporosis, as the vertebrae decrease in height, a person loses inches—sometimes five or six by 75 years of age. But though osteoporosis is the more common of the two bone disorders, an expert says that "osteoporosis and osteomalacia frequently coexist." And they may have the same cure. Vitamin D.

Researchers gave a concentrated form of vitamin D to seven women with osteoporosis, all of whom had suffered at least one fractured vertebra. During the year of treatment, the women had an improvement in their "calcium balance," so that "no further vertebral compression fractures were sustained during the treatment period" (*Clinical Research,* April, 1978).

So if you want to prevent your bones from softening, get outside as much as you can when the days are long and warm. And when you can't, get your "sunshine" from vitamin D.

Vitamin E for Nutrition That Starts at Skin Level

CHAPTER 12

Some vitamins not only help to keep us healthy on the inside, but come to our aid when we're hurt on the outside, too. Vitamin E is one of them. From patching up a nasty cut to keeping circulation flowing free and easy, vitamin E serves us in dozens of ways.

Patches Up Wounds as Good as New

"We've been using vitamin E here for years," said John Flanigan, M.D., a surgeon and director of the Enterostomal Therapy Unit at the Pottsville Hospital and Warne Clinic in Pennsylvania. Dr. Flanigan uses vitamin E ointment or oil in conjunction with oral supplements of E and zinc to promote the "secondary closure" of wounds.

A primary closure is when a cut is sewn up and it heals, explained Dr. Flanigan. A secondary closure means there is a gaping wound in which some skin has been lost and the tissue underneath is exposed. "Then I give patients the supplements and use vitamin E ointment or oil." Applying vitamin E helps the tiny red particles of new capillaries form on the surface of the wound to patch it together and heal.

"The tissue is fresher and the wound heals faster when vitamin E is applied to it," Dr. Flanigan told us. "But you have to have a good range of vitamin E systemically [inside the body] as well as locally." Healing time may be cut in half when vitamin E ointment or oil is used, he pointed out.

Dr. Flanigan said that vitamin E ointment and oil are effective on bedsores, too, and can be used in the home for minor first aid problems. They may be used for *any* minor cuts, abrasions and burns, he said, since "vitamin E is never going to hurt anybody." If you should fall and scrape yourself, for instance, Dr. Flanigan's advice is to thoroughly clean the wound, apply an antiseptic and then reach for the vitamin E. The wound should be recleaned and the vitamin E should be reapplied daily for the problem to heal quickly and safely, he said.

Cold Sores Disappear Fast

Vitamin E also has been reported successful in the treatment of cold sores (herpes simplex). At the health facilities of two industrial firms in Liverpool, England, an "unusually large number of patients" were seen suffering from cold sores, many of which were failing to respond well to standard treatment. Vitamin E capsules were handed out to the patients with instructions to apply the liquid contents to the lesions every four hours.

"The most striking results were: (a) quick and sustained relief of pain, and (b) early disappearance of the lesion," say the report's authors, who have treated at least 50 patients successfully with the method. "Now, as a matter of routine, patients with cold sores are given a capsule and are told how to apply the oil," they write (*British Dental Journal,* vol. 148, no. 11-1, 1980).

Natural Relief for Shingles

Related to cold sores—but much more agonizing—is an outbreak of shingles. After a bout of herpes zoster (the official name of this virus), the infection sometimes takes up residence in the spinal nerves, where it promptly goes into hibernation. You think it's gone forever, but it can wake up at any time and start multiplying. When that happens, the affected nerve becomes inflamed, and pain radiates all along its path. The herpes virus then passes down the nerve and multiplies again in the skin, causing clusters of sores—the "shingles"—to erupt on the chest, neck, lower back, forehead or eyes. Discomfort is extreme and may be constant or may come and go.

While there doesn't appear to be any definite way to ward off an attack of shingles, taking extra vitamin E may help ease the pain once the bug has struck. So says Richard Mihan, M.D., from the University of Southern California School of Medicine, who practices dermatology with Samuel Ayres, M.D.

Over a period of four years, Drs. Mihan and Ayres treated 13 patients with shingles with vitamin E, administered both orally (400 to 1,600 I.U. daily) and directly on the sores.

Eleven of the patients had had moderate to severe pain for

over six months. Seven of those had suffered for over 1 year, one for 13 years and one for 19 years. Yet after taking vitamin E, nine patients reported complete or almost complete control of pain. The two patients who had had the problem the longest were in this group. Of the remaining four patients, two were moderately improved (*Archives of Dermatology,* December, 1973).

A Balm for Breast Lumps

Vitamin E can often reduce noncancerous breast lumps— medically known as fibrocystic disease, cystic mastitis or mammary dysplasia. The slight rise in estrogen secretion by the ovaries that occurs about the middle of a woman's menstrual cycle seems to produce either fluid or solid cysts in some women's breasts. That results in unwelcome lumps the size of a grape or larger. And they can hurt!

Robert London, M.D., has found that vitamin E can often reduce not only the discomfort but also the size and number of breast cysts. As director of the Obstetric and Gynecologic Endocrinology Research Lab at Sinai Hospital in Baltimore, Dr. London has seen promising results from daily doses of 600 I.U. of vitamin E in 80 percent of one group of women studied. The nutrient seems to work by reversing the abnormal ratio of estrogen and progesterone circulating in a woman's body during her menstrual cycle. That change in hormone levels acts as an antidote to estrogen's disturbing effect of cyst formation in the breast.

Of course, should you unexpectedly discover a lump in your breast, you owe it to yourself to have your doctor check it out immediately on the outside chance it's more serious.

Your Circulation Deserves Vitamin E

Most of us probably take it for granted that our blood will flow through our veins as smoothly as water through pipes. But all too often arteries and veins clog up. And that's a lot more serious than a stopped-up water pipe. Narrowed blood vessels can lead to high blood pressure, angina, thrombophlebitis (inflammation of a vein associated with a blood clot)—or, worst of all, a heart attack.

But several researchers have insisted for some time that vitamin E may improve circulation and help prevent all those problems. One is R.V. Panganamala, Ph.D., of the department of physiological chemistry at Ohio State University School of Medicine in Columbus. Dr. Panganamala is conducting experiments with rabbits and rats to show how and why vitamin E is so crucial to the health of blood vessels.

Normally, blood flows through our veins without difficulty, Dr. Panganamala told us. But sometimes the vessel walls can narrow because blood platelets clump up against the inside of the vessel wall. (Platelets are tiny disk-shaped elements essential for clotting, or stopping the flow of blood in the event of a cut.)

"Anytime platelets stick together inside an intact blood vessel, it's a problem," explained Dr. Panganamala. "But that can happen when the platelets produce too much thromboxane, a substance that enhances their stickiness. It can also happen if the vessel wall doesn't produce enough prostacyclin. This chemical has the opposite effect on platelets—that is, it keeps them free-flowing and slippery.

"In our experiment," explained Dr. Panganamala, "we wanted to see what effect vitamin E had on those two chemicals. We used animals that were normal and healthy to begin with and divided them into two groups. One group received a diet high in vitamin E, while the other's diet had no vitamin E at all. After 10 to 12 weeks, we tested the levels of thromboxane and prostacyclin in the animals. We found that those deficient in vitamin E had significantly higher amounts of thromboxane [the chemical that makes platelets stickier], while at the same time, their vessels lost the capacity to produce prostacyclin [the chemical that keeps platelets apart].

"It's our current understanding that the proper ratio of thromboxane to prostacyclin is imperative if platelets are to move through the blood without aggregating [clumping up] at the wrong time. If the ratio's out of balance, there is a far greater chance of thrombosis [blood clots] to occur. Vitamin E helps keep those substances in precise, proper balance."

PREVENTS CLOGGED ARTERIES. But good circulation depends on more than smooth-flowing platelets. It's just as important to keep your blood vessels free of fatty buildup. And vitamin E can help again.

To prove this, researchers from the department of internal medicine at Kyoto University of Japan conducted a study to examine the effect of vitamin E on lipid peroxidation. (Lipid peroxides are produced when fat breaks down, or oxidizes, and are toxic to human and animal tissues. It's suspected that they accumulate in blood vessels and promote atherosclerosis and blood clots.) The researchers found that animals fed a diet deficient in vitamin E actually produced significantly more of these peroxides than a vitamin E-supplemented group.

The good news here is that the damages created by the vitamin E deficiency were reversible. The results support the possibility, cited by the researchers, that administration of vitamin E "could prevent and ameliorate vascular [vessel] damages" in some cases of heart disease (*Prostaglandins,* April, 1980).

J. C. Alexander, Ph.D., would agree. He's done his own experiments at the University of Guelph in Ontario, Canada, on the effects of vitamin E on oxidized fats.

"There is no doubt in my mind that vitamin E is a potent antioxidant and extremely important in maintaining a healthy circulatory system," he said. "Anyone who doesn't believe that is fooling himself."

CHEST PAINS REDUCED. Kaarlo Jaakkola, M.D., from the University of Jyvaskyla in Finland, also believes in vitamin E for tip-top circulation. He and his colleagues used vitamin E together with selenium to treat a group of 30 patients with heart disease. All the patients suffered from constant, moderate to severe chest pain—a sure sign of narrowed arteries—and needed large amounts of nitroglycerin and other medication to control the symptoms.

During the experimental period, one group of patients received daily doses of vitamin E and selenium while a second was given placebos. In the group treated with vitamin E and selenium, the first positive effects began to show up two weeks after the beginning of the treatment and the maximum effects after one to two months. With the majority of the treated patients, said the Finnish researchers, "the average daily usage of nitroglycerin decreased significantly" and they were able to walk farther without discomfort.

The researchers believe that vitamin E together with selenium has a beneficial effect on patients with heart disease, possibly because those nutrients help defend cells against lipid peroxides.

HELPS CONTROL CHOLESTEROL. While vitamin E is helping to reduce hazards such as lipid peroxides and overly sticky platelets, it's also helping to increase positive factors in your bloodstream. Specifically, there's evidence that it increases the level of high-density lipoprotein (HDL) cholesterol, the good kind of cholesterol, and decreases the level of low-density (LDL) or very-low-density (VLDL) cholesterol, the artery-clogging kind.

That point was demonstrated in an experiment conducted by William J. Hermann Jr., M.D., a pathologist at Memorial City General Hospital in Houston. He picked five people with average amounts of HDL cholesterol and five with low HDL levels (high risk for atherosclerosis) and placed them all on 600 I.U. of vitamin E per day. Within a few weeks, all five people with cholesterol problems increased their HDL levels between 220 and 483 percent.

Even four of the five people with average levels saw their HDL fractions rise as much as 237 percent (*American Journal of Clinical Pathology,* November, 1979).

The effect of the vitamin E appears to be a redistribution of cholesterol, said Dr. Hermann and his colleagues, elevating the HDL fraction and decreasing the VLDL part.

Dr. Hermann believes that the 15 to 50 units of vitamin E often found in multivitamin preparations probably aren't enough to have an effect on cholesterol metabolism. He suggests 400 I.U. as a good maintenance dose for the average person. He recommends higher doses—600 or 800 I.U.—at first for people with cholesterol imbalances.

High doses of vitamin E are not for everyone, though. Samuel Ayres, M.D., a Los Angeles dermatologist who's treated many people with nutritional therapy, told us that "people with high blood pressure, heart disease or diabetes should not take high levels of vitamin E at first. Vitamin E improves the tone of the heart muscle and a large dose too soon can make the blood pressure rise. Vitamin E also improves glycogen storage, so diabetics on insulin could develop an insulin shock reaction if they took too much vitamin E too soon. People with these conditions should not begin with any more than 100 I.U. of vitamin E a day. The dose may gradually be increased under a doctor's supervision."

A Shield against Pollution

OZONE. We already told you in chapter 10 that vitamin C can help protect your lungs from ozone, a major component of smog. But ozone does damage outside the lungs, too—it may harm red blood cells. And that's where vitamin E lends a hand.

When researchers at the University of Kentucky and the University of California at Davis fed rats a vitamin E-deficient diet and then exposed them to ozone, the rats' red blood cells showed significant damage. But cells of other animals fed supplemental vitamin E emerged unscathed (*Environmental Research,* June, 1979).

In another study, Daniel Menzel, Ph.D., a researcher at the Duke University Medical Center in Durham, North Carolina, continuously exposed three groups of mice to ozone. One group, however, received a large amount of vitamin E with its diet, another group got a smaller amount, and third group got no vitamin E. The group receiving the large amount of vitamin E survived an average of two weeks longer than the other groups (*Toxicology and Applied Pharmacology,* vol. 45, no. 1, 1978).

NITROGEN DIOXIDE (NO_2) was the focus of a second experiment, in which Dr. Menzel exposed two groups of mice to the pollutant, which is just as deadly as ozone. He gave one group a daily amount of vitamin E equivalent to what a person would get if he took a 100-I.U. supplement. The other group received the equivalent of 10 I.U. of vitamin E, the amount found in the average American's diet. After three months of exposure to nitrogen dioxide, both groups of mice had lung damage "very similar to what occurs in the early stages of human emphysema," said Dr. Menzel. *But the 100-I.U. mice had significantly less lung damage* (*Medical Tribune,* May 3, 1978).

Table 13
FOOD SOURCES OF VITAMIN E

Food	Portion	Vitamin E (international units)
Wheat germ oil	1 tablespoon	37.2
Sunflower seeds	¼ cup	26.8
Wheat germ, raw	½ cup	12.8
Sunflower seed oil	1 tablespoon	12.7
Almonds	¼ cup	12.7
Pecans, halves	¼ cup	12.5
Hazelnuts	¼ cup	12.0
Safflower oil	1 tablespoon	7.9
Peanuts	¼ cup	4.9
Corn oil	1 tablespoon	4.8
Cod-liver oil	1 tablespoon	3.9
Peanut butter	2 tablespoons	3.8
Corn oil margarine	1 tablespoon	3.6
Soybean oil	1 tablespoon	3.5
Peanut oil	1 tablespoon	3.4
Lobster	3 ounces	2.3
Salmon steak	3 ounces	2.0

SOURCES: Adapted from
"Vitamin E Content of Foods," by P. J. McLaughlin and John L. Weihrauch, *Journal of the American Dietetic Association,* December, 1979.
Nutritive Value of American Foods in Common Units, Agriculture Handbook No. 456, by Catherine F. Adams (Washington, D.C.: Agricultural Research Service, U.S. Department of Agriculture, 1975).
McCance and Widdowson's The Composition of Foods, by A. A. Paul and D. A. T. Southgate (Elsevier/North-Holland Biomedical, 1978).

To protect his own health, Dr. Menzel takes 200 I.U. of vitamin E every day. "A study I'm now completing may show if a higher amount is needed," he said. "But 200 I.U. should help protect the body from the stress of air pollution." (For more on our nutritional defense against pollution, see the chapters on vitamin A and vitamin C.)

Whole Foods Are Vitamin E Foods

To get the most vitamin E in your diet, eat whole foods like grains and avoid processed and refined foods. Canned and frozen foods lose up to 65 percent of their vitamin E. Nuts, a notably good source, lose up to 80 percent of their vitamin E when roasted. Oils, too, provide plenty of vitamin E—unless they're hydrogenated. (See table 13 for a list of foods that supply significant amounts of vitamin E.)

But if you want foolproof insurance, take the advice of some of the scientists we talked to and take a supplement. With vitamin E, you can't go wrong.

Your Foundation Needs Vitamin K

13

What vitamin is found in such large quantities in nature, and required in such small amounts by the body, that deficiencies were always thought to be rare? Most people haven't even heard of it. It's not commonly available in supplemental form, because we apparently need no more of it than is available in a good, sensible diet. And part of our supply of the vitamin is produced in the body itself, by bacteria in the intestinal tract.

Sounds like the ultimate wallflower nutrient, doesn't it, so taken for granted that most people don't even know it exists. There is such a thing as vitamin K, though, and we'd all be in deep trouble without it.

Vitamin K is required for the production of a number of coagulation factors, substances in the blood which are essential for normal blood clotting. Nosebleeds, bleeding in the intestines and stomach, and blood in the urine are all common in vitamin K deficiency. Bleeding may occur within the brain, and the deficiency can result in death.

But if vitamin K deficiency is so rare, what's the problem? Scientists used to believe there was no problem at all, but now they're not so sure. Until a few years ago, the only role vitamin K was known to play in maintaining good health was its assurance of proper blood clotting. And people were certainly not bleeding to death because of vitamin K deficiencies. Indeed, it was hard to find even minor problems caused by a lack of vitamin K.

Your Bones Depend on Vitamin K, Too

Now, however, a body of evidence is building which indicates
76 that vitamin K may do more than promote coagulation. Recent

research at Harvard University, the University of California at San Diego, and other scientific centers suggests that vitamin K is necessary for the maintenance of healthy bones as well. There is evidence, a spokesperson for the Harvard research team told us, that slight vitamin K deficiencies in older people may be contributing to the degeneration of bone so common at that time of life.

As we grow older, and particularly as women undergo menopause, something happens to disrupt the healthy turnover of bone. A condition called osteoporosis may set in, causing loss of bone mass, and increasing fragility of the bones. The condition affects three out of every four women after menopause, resulting in a frightening increase in broken bones. By the age of 90, one woman out of every five fractures a hip, and one of every six of those women dies within three months of the injury. Studies have already shown that extra calcium and vitamin D in the diet can help prevent osteoporosis.

But scientists in Japan have also used vitamin K to reduce the loss of calcium from the bones that occurs in osteoporosis.

"The Japanese scientists looked at three osteoporosis patients. In the three women, vitamin K reduced calcium loss in the bone by 18 percent in one patient, 50 percent in another and 21 percent in the third" the Harvard researcher told us.

That vitamin K could become a widely used therapy to fight osteoporosis is a tantalizing possibility, and the Harvard scientist told us there are plenty of other indications that such therapy could help.

"Osteoporosis occurs mainly in older people. Those people often eat soft, bland foods and fail to eat enough green vegetables, which are rich in vitamin K. Studies in England have shown that older people are commonly slightly vitamin K deficient, in that their blood coagulation activity is slightly reduced. Older people also often take mineral oil as a laxative, which interferes with the way vitamin K is absorbed into the body."

Other drugs which older people are more likely to use— including anticoagulants, antibiotics and cholestyramine, a drug used to lower cholesterol levels in the blood—may all contribute to vitamin K deficiency.

Help Yourself to Vitamin K-Rich Greens

How can you be sure to get enough of the nutrient?

"Diets containing plenty of fresh green vegetables will provide adequate vitamin K," the Harvard spokesperson said. Broccoli, cabbage, lettuce, turnip greens and spinach are all good sources. (See table 14.)

And though no one knows for sure *exactly* how much vitamin K the average adult needs, there have been some estimates.

The National Research Council, which draws up the Recommended Dietary Allowances for nutrients used by the government, does not have an official RDA for vitamin K, but they do make a ball-park guess. They say the average adult needs between 70 and 140 micrograms of K each day. That's not too difficult. For example, to get 140 micrograms of vitamin K, you would have to eat about 2½ ounces of broccoli. (You'd probably be better off with a bit more vitamin K, especially if you're over 60 or so.) Sounds like a very sensible approach indeed to avoiding what could be very nasty health problems.

Table 14
FOOD SOURCES OF VITAMIN K

Food	Portion	Vitamin K (micrograms)
Turnip greens, cooked	½ cup	471
Broccoli, cooked	1 medium stalk	360
Cabbage, shredded, cooked	½ cup	91
Beef liver	3 ounces	78
Lettuce, chopped	1 cup packed	71
Spinach, raw, chopped	1 cup packed	49
Asparagus	4 medium spears	34
Cheese	2 ounces	20
Watercress, finely chopped	¼ cup	18
Peas	½ cup	15
Green beans	½ cup	9
Milk	1 cup	7

SOURCES: Adapted from
Modern Nutrition in Health and Disease, by Robert S. Goodhart and Maurice E. Shills (Philadelphia: Lea & Febiger, 1980).
Nutritive Value of American Foods in Common Units, Agriculture Handbook No. 456, by Catherine F. Adams (Washington, D.C.: Agricultural Research Service, U.S. Department of Agriculture, 1975).
Composition of Foods: Dairy and Egg Products, Agriculture Handbook No. 8-1, by Consumer and Food Economics Institute (Washington, D.C.: Agricultural Research Service, U.S. Department of Agriculture, 1976).

How Much Do You Need? A Guide to Vitamin Supplementation

CHAPTER 14

No one can say what level of supplementation is exactly right for you. With changes occurring almost continuously in our bodies, our diets and our environments—not to mention changes in nutritional science itself—it is just not possible to be terribly precise.

Still, we all need some general guidelines that will put us on the right track, if not right on the mark, so far as supplements are concerned. That's what we're trying to provide here.

Please keep in mind the following:

1. These guidelines are not specific recommendations, but rather general, informational statements which inevitably reflect a certain degree of opinion as well as current research.

2. For each nutrient, read the paragraph of descriptive statements accompanying the various amounts. *Find the paragraph which most closely describes you.* It is not necessary, or in some cases even possible, for each sentence in the paragraph to describe you specifically. Go with the one that, *overall,* seems most applicable.

3. If you have a symptom that suggests a deficiency or special need for one B vitamin, chances are you're deficient in another. The B vitamins work together, so if you take a larger amount of a single B vitamin, make sure you also take a supplement that contains the entire B complex.

4. Don't try to use the information here to pinpoint nutritional causes of symptoms. Analyzing serious symptoms is your doctor's job.

Vitamin A

5,000 I.U. Your diet regularly includes liver, carrots, broccoli, apricots, sweet potatoes and spinach. You are generally in excellent **79**

health, your resistance is very high, and the environment in which you live is low in pollutants. Naturally, you are not a smoker and never have been. Nor are there any smokers in your household. There is nothing in your family history that makes you particularly concerned about cancer.

10,000 I.U. You eat vitamin A-rich foods such as liver, carrots and sweet potatoes occasionally, but they're not on your menu every day. Your health is better than average, but you are not invulnerable, and you know that when your resistance gets low, you tend to become ill, perhaps with upper respiratory symptoms. Skin problems are not unknown to you. You are exposed to an average amount of pollution from various sources.

25,000 I.U. Occasionally, you notice patches of dry, bumpy skin on your legs or arms. Not dry and flaky, but dry and *bumpy*. Recently you may have been involved in a serious health crisis, such as surgery, an injury, burn or other problem that had you out of circulation for more than just a few days. Your vision, especially at dusk, is not what it could be. Foods such as liver, spinach and carrots have been known to appear on your dining room table, but they are hardly fixtures.

Note: *Normally, supplements of vitamin A should not exceed about 50,000 I.U. per day. Very large amounts—usually well over 100,000 I.U. per day—can cause symptoms of toxicity, such as dry skin and loss of appetite. The amounts mentioned in this guide, however, are perfectly safe for adults.*

Thiamine (Vitamin B$_1$)
5 MILLIGRAMS. You're practically famous for your perpetual good mood and unflagging energy. Your diet regularly includes brewer's yeast, wheat germ, whole grain products, liver and sunflower seeds.

10 MILLIGRAMS. You're generally a frisky sort, even though you aren't necessarily ready to conquer the world at the dawn of each and every day. There are times when you wish your nerves were better behaved, and you sometimes think you drink too much coffee or tea for your own good. Your diet is average.

25 MILLIGRAMS. Your nerves are definitely in a state, and you may be suffering from depression, loss of appetite or similar emotional and neurological problems. Your energy levels are at best undependable, as is your memory. Possibly you are in your retirement years, when absorption of thiamine—as well as other B vitamins—is very much reduced.

Riboflavin (Vitamin B₂)

5 MILLIGRAMS. You're a great one for dairy foods like milk and cheese. Almonds, broccoli, liver and other riboflavin-rich foods appear in your daily fare. Your eyes are clear and bright and the skin around your mouth is perfectly smooth—except when you smile, which you do frequently.

10 MILLIGRAMS. You don't care for milk and liver, cheese and eggs have too much cholesterol for you, and wild rice and asparagus are too expensive. So you don't get that much riboflavin in your diet except from your whole grain bread. You are also getting up there in years.

25 MILLIGRAMS. If you look in the mirror carefully, you will see small cracks around your mouth, or your tongue may be smooth and purplish. Your eyes may burn, itch, be abnormally sensitive to bright light, or simply feel worn out. You may feel depressed. You are no spring chicken.

Niacin

10 MILLIGRAMS. Your diet regularly includes fish, beans, organ meats, peanuts, poultry, whole wheat products and brewer's yeast. Or at least half of those foods. Your disposition is strictly blue sky. The only time you are irritable is when enemy tanks invade your neighborhood.

25 MILLIGRAMS. Your diet is nothing to brag about, particularly, and occasionally you wonder if there is some reason why it's becoming so difficult for you to fall asleep. Or if your headaches have some peculiar origin.

50 MILLIGRAMS. Your nerves and your personality are definitely not what they used to be and not what your friends or family would like them to be. You may have thought about visiting a psychologist or psychiatrist and you would be grateful if something could be done about your insomnia.

Vitamin B₆ (Pyridoxine)

5 MILLIGRAMS. You practically radiate good health, and your positive, energetic attitude is reflected in your intelligently varied diet, which includes brown rice, salmon, liver, bananas and, of course, whole grains.

10 MILLIGRAMS. You certainly aren't sick, but you sometimes wonder why your skin isn't better, or why your nerves aren't calmer. You may tend to retain a lot of fluid before your menstrual periods.

50 MILLIGRAMS. Your monthly periods cause you considerable distress, not only because of fluid retention, but because of emotional problems at that time—or perhaps *all* the time. Possibly you are on birth control pills. Life is looking more and more like an ordeal.

Vitamin B$_{12}$ (Cobalamin)

5 MICROGRAMS. You are healthy, energetic, haven't yet reached retirement age, and you regularly eat animal foods such as meat, fish or chicken.

10 MICROGRAMS. You've passed your sixtieth birthday and your ability to absorb this vitamin in a useful form may be on the wane.

25 MICROGRAMS. Lately, your energy level and possibly your nerves just haven't been up to snuff. Possibly you've been ill or had surgery. You may be a strict vegan, one who avoids all animal-source foods. These symptoms may well be serious enough to suggest a thorough medical evaluation.

Folate

400 MICROGRAMS. You eat a lot of raw green vegetables such as broccoli, romaine lettuce and brussels sprouts. You're a liver lover from way back, and you eat it with onions. You are full of energy and retirement is something that's far in the future.

400 TO 800 MICROGRAMS. You must remind yourself that you should eat raw green vegetables more frequently, and you wish you were able to work out a way to eat beans, beets, broccoli and brewer's yeast more often than you do. Your health is about average. If you're a woman, you're either pregnant, nursing, or taking oral contraceptives.

800 TO 2,000 MICROGRAMS. Lately, you feel as though you've been under considerable emotional stress, and you haven't been able to handle it as well as you should. Your nerves in general have been in such a state that you have given serious consideration to seeking some kind of help, whether it be medical, psychological or even nutritional. You are over 70 years of age and your absorption, therefore, of folate is likely to be impaired. Possibly, you have recently undergone surgery. Your doctor may have reason to believe you have folate deficiency anemia which causes, among other things, inflammation of the tongue, digestive problems and diarrhea. (When taking folate supplements, always take vitamin B$_{12}$ with them.)

Vitamin C

100 MILLIGRAMS. You can hardly remember the last time you were ill. Your health is excellent, and your gums are clear, firm and never bleed. Your daily diet includes generous measures of such vitamin C-rich foods as broccoli, cabbage, melons, citrus fruits and green peppers.

500 MILLIGRAMS. You feel that your resistance must be maintained at a high level in order to keep you feeling your best. There may be some chronic health problem or stress in your life, such as a bad back, allergies or exposure to cigarette smoke. Your diet is not bad by a long shot, but does not supply the amount of ascorbic acid you feel you should get.

2,000 MILLIGRAMS. You are definitely susceptible to stresses such as infection, pain or skin problems. Possibly you are recovering from surgery, an injury or any other serious bout with illness. In the past, you have noticed that injury or surgical incisions seem to heal very slowly. Your diet could be better, but it is difficult for you to eat raw foods, high in vitamin C, because they tend to make your gums bleed. You may want to step down to a lower level of vitamin C supplementation when the health problem or crisis you are now undergoing disappears.

Vitamin D

0 TO 200 I.U. You live in an area where the sun shines strong and bright, such as Florida or southern California. What's more, you move around quite a bit outdoors, so that sunlight strikes your body, causing your system to manufacture its own vitamin D. If you have a year-round tan, you probably don't need any supplemental vitamin D at all.

400 I.U. You live in an area such as Pennsylvania or the state of Washington, where a beautiful sunshiny day is a real event. You are not a big drinker of milk, which is fortified with vitamin D, usually at the rate of about 400 I.U. per quart. Occasionally, however, you do eat fish containing vitamin D, such as herring, mackerel, salmon, sardines and tuna.

800 I.U. You probably live in the northern United States, Canada or England, where, except for a few weeks in the middle of summer, intense sunshine may be as rare as rainbows. What's more, for one reason or another, you do not get very much exercise outdoors. Possibly you have had a problem with your bones, suffering a fracture or pain. Although a physician may recommend considerably higher supplements, you should not ordinarily take more than this amount on your own each day, as vitamin D tends to accumulate in the body, and very large amounts (usually many thousands of I.U.) can become toxic.

Vitamin E

100 I.U. You are relatively young, in fine health, and you live in an exceptionally clean area, where there is remarkably little pollution.

400 I.U. You may have a health condition which may be prevented or improved with vitamin E, such as intermittent claudication (cramping of the calf on walking), or any one of a number of skin problems. The air you breathe, the water you drink, and possibly the food you eat contain the usual amount of pollutants found in our modern world. Your diet contains a substantial amount of polyunsaturated fats, such as corn oil.

600 I.U. You may be concerned about a circulation problem and feel that the beneficial effect of vitamin E on blood elements is something that you want to take advantage of in full measure.

YOUR PERSONAL SUPPLEMENT PROFILE

Circle the amounts best for you as determined in this chapter.

Vitamin	Units	Amounts		
Vitamin A	I.U.	5,000	10,000	25,000
Thiamine (B_1)	milligrams	5	10	25
Riboflavin (B_2)	milligrams	5	10	25
Niacin	milligrams	10	25	50
B_6 (pyridoxine)	milligrams	5	10	50
B_{12} (cobalamin)	micrograms	5	10	25
Folate	micrograms	400	400-800	800-2,000
Vitamin C	milligrams	100	500	2,000
Vitamin D	I.U.	0-200	400	800
Vitamin E	I.U.	100	400	600

Appendix:
Drug–Vitamin Interactions

The following table highlights a few common drug-vitamin interactions. However, if you are taking *any* medication, listed here or not, it's important that you consult your doctor about its interaction with vitamins.

Because of space limitations, only categories or common names of drugs are given. Brand names are not. Therefore, be sure to ask your pharmacist for both the generic name of your medication and its type if the information on its label doesn't allow you to match the drug to this chart.

These drugs:	may interact with these vitamins:	so that:
antacids	thiamine	thiamine is destroyed when antacids are taken at mealtime. Even if you take supplements, antacids may cancel them out if taken at the same time.
antibiotics	vitamin C	the urine becomes more acidic and kidney stones may develop.
	vitamin K	a vitamin K deficiency may result.

(continued)

SOURCES: Adapted from
Drug-Induced Nutritional Deficiencies, by Daphne A. Roe (Westport, Conn.: Avi, 1976).
The People's Pharmacy — 2, by Joe Graedon with Teresa Graedon (New York: Avon, 1980).
The Woman's Encyclopedia of Health and Natural Healing, by Emrika Padus (Emmaus, Pa.: Rodale Press, 1981).

These drugs:	may interact with these vitamins:	so that:
anticoagulants	vitamin C	the drugs' blood-thinning effect may be altered. This is a controversial issue so play it safe and have your blood clotting time checked if you start or stop large doses of vitamin C.
	vitamin E	the blood-thinning action of these drugs may be too strong.
	vitamin K	the blood-thinning action of these drugs is diminished. Too many vitamin K-rich vegetables can reverse the anticoagulant effect.
anticonvulsants	vitamin C	the sedative effect of these drugs is enhanced.
	vitamin D	vitamin D may be depleted.
	folate	the anticonvulsant drug phenytoin depletes the body of folate.
aspirin	vitamin C	more of the vitamin and less of the aspirin is excreted in the urine. As a result, aspirin's effect is increased.
	folate	folic acid anemia (the formation of abnormally large red blood cells) may result in people who take aspirin in high doses over a long period of time.
cholestyramine	vitamin A, B_{12}, D, K	these vitamins are not absorbed very well.
clofibrate	vitamin B_{12}	vitamin B_{12} absorption may be reduced.
laxatives containing phosphates	vitamin D	regular laxative use can deplete body calcium and interfere with vitamin D utilization.

These drugs:	may interact with these vitamins:	so that:
levodopa	vitamin B_6	vitamin B_6 speeds the breakdown of levodopa, reducing the drug's effectiveness.
methotrexate	folate	the drug is antagonistic to folate and may produce anemia.
	riboflavin	the effectiveness of this anticancer drug may be reduced.
oral contraceptives	vitamin B_6	the need for vitamin B_6 is increased.
	vitamin C	the body is depleted of vitamin C.
	vitamin E	blood levels of vitamin E may drop.
	folate	the need for folate is increased.
penicillamine	vitamin B_6	a vitamin B_6 deficiency can develop.
potassium chloride	vitamin B_{12}	the vitamin is poorly absorbed.
sulfa drugs	vitamin C	kidney stones could develop because vitamin C makes the urine more acidic.
	PABA	the drugs are less effective.

Index